AF421889

UNLOCK YOUR BEAUTY & GLOW FROM WITHIN

Mrs. Hang Hoang
Unlock Your Beauty & Glow From Within

All rights reserved
Copyright © 2025 by Mrs. Hang Hoang

No part of this publication may be reproduced, distributed, or transmitted in any form or by any means, including photocopying, recording, or other electronic or mechanical methods, without the prior written permission of the publisher, except in the case of brief quotations embodied in critical reviews and certain other noncommercial uses permitted by copyright law.

Published by Spines
ISBN 979-8-89691-428-0

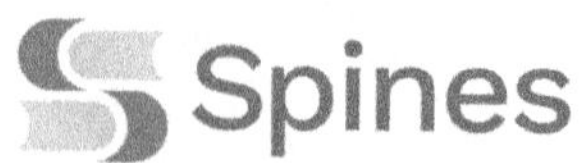

UNLOCK YOUR BEAUTY & GLOW FROM WITHIN

A HOLISTIC GUIDE TO HEALTH, CONFIDENCE & RADIANCE

MRS. HANG HOANG

CONTENTS

INTRODUCTION

Are you ready to reclaim your glow, confidence, and vitality? Unlock Your Beauty & Glow From Within is your ultimate guide to a holistic approach to health, wellness, and beauty—a journey that goes beyond skin deep.

In today's fast-paced world, the pressures of modern life often cloud our sense of self-worth and well-being. This book offers a refreshing perspective, blending time-tested natural remedies with contemporary insights to help you reconnect with your inner and outer radiance. From understanding the mind-beauty connection and managing hormonal changes to embracing aging with grace and navigating chronic conditions, this guide provides practical, transformative strategies for every stage of life.

Discover how to:

- Revitalize your skin, hair, and overall health with mindful, organic practices.
- Unlock ancient beauty secrets for lasting confidence and natural radiance.
- Embrace self-care rituals that nurture both body and soul.

With actionable steps, powerful affirmations, and heartfelt advice, this book empowers you to redefine beauty on your own terms—affirming that true beauty starts from within.

Your transformation begins here. Open the pages and step into a life where health, wellness, and beauty come together to create a more radiant, empowered you.

Your glow is waiting—are you ready to claim it?

CHAPTER 1
FROM STRUGGLES TO STRENGTH
MY PATH TO HOLISTIC LIVING

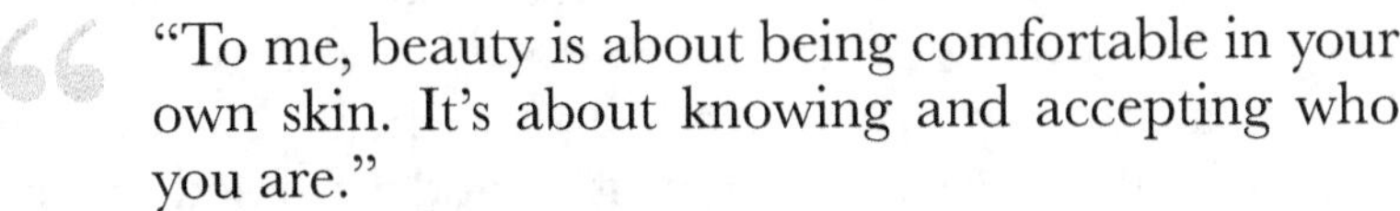

"To me, beauty is about being comfortable in your own skin. It's about knowing and accepting who you are."

— Ellen DeGeneres

A LIFE OF EARLY CHALLENGES AND RESILIENCE

When I was two months old, my family's life changed dramatically. I wouldn't call it rough at the time since all I could do was eat and sleep. I had no awareness of the world around me. But as I grew older, the significance of those early moments began to unfold. During my childhood, Vietnam had strict policies regarding childbirth, particularly for teachers like my parents. They were not allowed to have children too close in age. As a result, my parents faced disciplinary action from the government and were forced to relocate to a very remote area in the mountains.

Our living conditions were far from favorable. My father told me that he had to ride 11 miles with my mother sitting behind him on his bike, holding me as a newborn while my 14-month-old sister sat in the front. Although I was oblivious to our hardships, I was already part of the struggles my family endured.

It was not until I was four years old that I began to understand how dire our situation was. Let me paint a vivid picture: here we were, a family of four, packed into a dingy, old studio—so small that we could hear each other breathe. Our "apartment" was in an isolated area near a school, surrounded by similar homes. The roof was made of rice straw. Despite both of my parents being teachers, they earned very little, and supporting the family was difficult. To make ends meet, my parents began farming peanuts and cultivating unused land. My sister and I started working on the farm at the ages of six and five.

Looking back, I am immensely proud of my family and myself for our resilience under such tough circumstances. Today, as a mother of three young children, I nurture and ensure that my kids' needs are always met. It feels surreal when I think about how, at five and six years old, my sister and I worked on the farm—alone. I remember a time when a man on a bike called out to us while we worked and offered us candy. Even now, I get goosebumps thinking about it. What if that man had bad intentions? Fortunately, nothing happened, and he simply gave us candy and went on his way. But now, as a mother, the thought of my own children living the life I did terrifies me.

When I turned nine, my parents were notified by the government that we could return to our hometown. My father was tasked with moving all our belongings while my mother stayed behind to care for my sick sister and newborn brother. I remember wondering why my father did not ask for help from our relatives. His simple answer? They were too busy. So, together, we set off, pushing a wagon piled high with everything we owned. We walked through the night, stopping only to rest along the side of the road, and by morning, we were close to home. But by then, I had fallen ill, and an acquaintance offered to take me to my grandfather's house until I recovered.

I also wonder why my father chose to travel at night instead of during the day. Perhaps it was a matter of shame—maybe he did not want others to see our poverty and witness a teacher's family in such dire straits.

Eventually, we all moved back into our old home, and I regained my health. However, we continued farming to support the family, switching from peanuts to growing rice. My sister and I continued to work in the fields, and I experienced many unforgettable moments during those years.

You might be wondering: "Why am I sharing my story in a book about health and beauty?" By sharing my journey, I hope to inspire you to overcome the barriers and challenges you face in your life.

UNPREDICTABLE CHALLENGES: LESSONS IN COURAGE AND FAMILY STRENGTH

One of the greatest challenges we faced as farmers was Vietnam's unpredictable weather. We used to dry rice seeds in the front yard after harvesting, but Vietnam often experiences sudden thunderstorms, which could ruin our crops. Whenever the clouds began to darken, it was a race against time to get all of our rice seeds inside the house before the rain hit. These moments helped me hone my quick-thinking skills and my ability to solve problems before they escalated.

But sometimes, no matter how hard you try, life throws you a storm you simply cannot outrun. During my childhood, Vietnam experienced the worst flood of the century. Initially, my father stayed behind after getting my mother, my siblings, and me onto a boat to seek refuge at my grandparents' house. He tried to protect our home by moving everything he could to higher ground, hoping to salvage some of our belongings. But he did not expect the water to rise so fast. Eventually, the house became fully submerged.

I vividly remember sitting in the boat, soaked from head to toe, faint with hunger and exhaustion. Worst of all, we had no word from my father. Hours turned into days, and the fear that he might have been swept away in the flood gripped us. It was the scariest time of my life—I still get goosebumps writing about it now. We could not sleep, consumed with worry, and we cried the entire night, thinking he might be gone. Outside, the streets had turned into rivers of brown water filled with debris—dead animals, trees, and remnants of people's homes. Those were the gloomiest, most terrifying days I've ever lived through.

Two days felt like an eternity. Then, finally, our nightmare ended. My father was alive! Villagers rescued him by boat, and I leapt up and down, overwhelmed with joy. That evening, we all gathered around him as he recounted his near-death experience. He had been the last to evacuate, and by the time he left the house, the water was too strong for a regular boat. He and the other villagers had to take shelter in a public building, which was already showing signs of collapse. Miraculously, they were rescued by a city boat just before the building gave way. Truly, that flood taught me to face life's storms with faith and determination, knowing that even in the darkest moments, there's a chance for light.

A NEW CHAPTER: FINDING MY PATH IN AMERICA

My life took a dramatic turn when I came to America by myself at the age of 17. It was a leap into the unknown, filled with hope and uncertainty. I'm deeply grateful to God for this opportunity and to my American host family, who embraced me as one of their own. Though I stayed with them for only a short time, their simple and intentional way of living left an indelible mark on me.

They lived with a focus on non-materialistic values, prioritizing health, relationships, and inner contentment over external appearances. This shaped my understanding of what true beauty really means. Seeing how naturally happy and radiant my American mother and sisters were taught me a lesson I've carried ever since: **outer beauty is simply a reflection of inner self-worth.** They didn't chase after glamour or obsess over cosmetics, yet their kindness and authenticity made them truly beautiful.

LESSONS IN TRUE BEAUTY: INNER WORTH REFLECTS OUTER RADIANCE

As I reflect on my journey, I realize how much life's challenges have refined me. They've taught me to treasure not just outward beauty but the strength, resilience, and purpose that lie within. True beauty isn't about meeting external standards —it's about living authentically and embracing who you are at your core.

A JOURNEY INTO SUSTAINABLE LIVING AND HOLISTIC HEALTH

The journey I've walked—marked by its share of joys and struggles—has laid the foundation for a life filled with purpose and gratitude. Even during the toughest times, the lessons my parents instilled in me stood as a guiding light. They taught me to find abundance in simplicity and to cherish the natural world as a source of strength and inspiration.

Our modest way of living wasn't about sacrifice—it was about thriving with the gifts nature offers. Those simple, grounded days taught me to see nature not just as a backdrop to life but as a partner in health and well-being. My connection to nature isn't just a preference; it's a principle that guides my daily choices. I've embraced a holistic lifestyle because I truly believe that Mother Nature provides everything we need to flourish— health, beauty, and balance.

TURNING PASSION INTO PURPOSE

This belief led me to participate in the Mrs. California Earth pageant—a platform that celebrates sustainability, empowerment, and the natural world. As a titleholder, I found a voice to share my passion for holistic living and for helping women recognize their worth. This book grew out of that passion, a way to dedicate my journey and knowledge to women everywhere.

For me, beauty is far more than what we see in the mirror. It's about nurturing a healthy body, a resilient mind, and a fulfilled spirit. When these elements come together in harmony, they radiate confidence, joy, and strength. As women, we carry so much on our shoulders—our families, our work, our dreams—but we also deserve to care for ourselves, to thrive, and to feel truly beautiful, inside and out.

AN INVITATION TO HOLISTIC LIVING

In this chapter, I've shared a glimpse of my life—the ups and downs that shaped me into who I am today. Life hasn't always been easy, but every challenge taught me resilience and helped me grow. By sharing my story, my hope is to encourage you to face your own obstacles with courage and grace and to remind you that you are strong, you are worthy, and you are beautiful.

As you turn the pages of this book, we'll dive into a holistic approach to beauty and wellness. Together, we'll explore how physical health supports radiant skin, how mental well-being fosters resilience, and how lifestyle choices empower us to lead vibrant, joyful lives. We'll discuss topics like mental health, gut health, hormonal changes, weight loss, and self-care. We'll also address important health concerns such as breast and cervical cancer and delve into the benefits of practices like aromatherapy, music therapy, embracing AI's influence on modern women's lifestyles, and many more helpful topics.

This isn't just a book—it's an invitation to transform how you see yourself and how you live your life. It's about building confidence, prioritizing your well-being, and embracing the beauty that is uniquely yours. Together, let's take this journey of self-discovery, empowerment, and holistic living. You deserve it, and it starts now. Let's begin.

CHAPTER 2

UNFILTERED CONFIDENCE: REDEFINING BEAUTY IN THE AGE OF SOCIAL MEDIA

THE HIDDEN COST OF FILTERS AND HOW TO RECLAIM YOUR TRUE BEAUTY

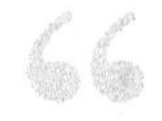 "Be your own kind of beautiful."

— Unknown

On a scale of 1 to 10, how beautiful does social media make you feel? Take a moment to think about this as you read on. Reflect on how the endless scroll through apps and feeds has shaped your perception of beauty, your self-worth, and even the way you define confidence.

THE ALLURE OF PERFECTION: HOW SOCIAL MEDIA SHAPES OUR PERCEPTION OF BEAUTY

Chances are, your phone is within arm's reach right now. In the past hour, you might have found yourself scrolling through **Instagram, TikTok, Snapchat, or Facebook**, casually flipping through a sea of posts. Maybe you've paused on a few: influencers showing off perfectly styled outfits, celebrities flaunting glowing skin, or even friends capturing what looks like an effortless "good hair day." Each image is meticulously curated, filtered, and captioned to perfection.

Now, let's dig a little deeper. Picture yourself scrolling through these perfectly polished posts. You stop to admire stunning models with their flawless outfits and airbrushed complexions. What comes to mind? Do you feel inspired, motivated to try a new style or skincare product? Or does that familiar wave of comparison wash over you—the feeling that you'll never measure up to this unattainable standard of beauty?

THE RISE OF BEAUTY FILTERS AND AI MANIPULATION

Social media platforms like **Instagram, Snapchat, and Facebook** thrive on visuals, making beauty filters one of their most popular features. With just a swipe, these filters can smooth your skin, contour your cheekbones, brighten your eyes, or even reshape your entire face. While they might seem like harmless fun, their influence runs deeper, leading to what experts now call Snapchat dysmorphia—a growing obsession with looking like an idealized, filtered version of yourself.

But filters are no longer just about airbrushing your skin or enhancing your eyes. AI technology has taken it to a whole new level, allowing users to completely alter their bodies at the tap of a finger. Today, apps integrated into **Instagram, Facebook, and Snapchat** can slim waists, add curves, make hair appear fuller, or even tweak your facial structure to resemble an entirely different person. These aren't minor touch-ups; they're complete reconstructions of reality—creating a version of yourself that doesn't actually exist.

What's troubling is that this shift is reshaping how we see ourselves and each other. How often do we compare our unfiltered reflections to these AI-altered images and feel like we're falling short? It's not just about chasing perfection—it's about chasing something that isn't even real.

THE TRAP OF TRENDS: WHY CHASING BEAUTY STANDARDS NEVER ENDS

Beauty trends have always evolved, but the speed and intensity of modern trends are truly next level. Remember when heavy contouring was all the rage, and suddenly, everyone switched to the dewy, "glass skin" look? Or when bold, dramatic makeup was everywhere, only to be replaced by minimalist, barely-there beauty? Social media has turned these trends into a revolving door—one day it's full glam, the next it's "clean girl" aesthetic.

The challenge isn't just the rapid pace of these trends but the pressure they create. With every swipe, you're met with a new standard, a new ideal to chase. Suddenly, it feels like what worked for you yesterday isn't "enough" today. It's exhausting trying to keep up when the goalposts keep moving.

And let's talk about the "natural beauty" trend for a moment. The polished yet effortless look seems so achievable—until you realize it often takes hours of preparation and a curated arsenal of expensive products. It's no wonder so many of us feel like we're falling short.

Social media, powered by AI tools, has only made this cycle more intense. Filters can give you instant glassy skin, exaggerated cheekbones, or the perfect eyeliner flick, but they also create an unattainable version of beauty. The problem is that these trends are fleeting, leaving women caught in a never-ending chase that can feel overwhelming and unachievable.

But here's the truth: beauty doesn't have an expiration date, and it certainly doesn't need to follow every trend. Instead of chasing the ever-changing standards, wouldn't it feel better to define beauty on your own terms?

WHY THIS MATTERS: THE EMOTIONAL IMPACT OF UNREALISTIC STANDARDS

Let's be honest—beauty trends, AI filters, and perfectly curated social media feeds can make any of us feel like we're falling short. I know because I've been there. Scrolling through **Instagram** or **Facebook**, I've caught myself gazing at picture-perfect posts, thinking, Wow, I wish my life looked like that. Those flawless photos of sparkling kitchens, romantic vacations, or glowing skin can stir up this nagging feeling of, Am I doing enough?

The truth is, beauty isn't about chasing some ever-changing, unattainable ideal. It's about embracing your own story, your own light, and finding confidence in who you are without the filters. Trends come and go, but the real you—authentic, unfiltered, and beautifully imperfect—is what truly matters.

By taking a step back and recognizing the influence of AI, beauty filters, and social media trends, we reclaim the power to see our worth beyond these illusions. Let's stop chasing fleeting perfection and start celebrating the beauty that's already within us.

BREAKING FREE: PRACTICAL WAYS TO RECLAIM YOUR CONFIDENCE

If you've ever found yourself stuck in the scroll, comparing your real life to someone's highlight reel, here's what's helped me—and it might work for you too:

1. **Take a Social Media Detox**: I know it's easier said than done, but taking a break can be a game-changer. There have been times when I've felt overwhelmed by all the perfect posts on **Instagram** or **Snapchat**, so I simply deleted the app for a week. Honestly, it was like a breath of fresh air. Without constant reminders of what I "should" be, I could focus on what I already have and feel grateful for it.

2. **Set Limits and Stick to Them**: If deleting isn't your thing (I get it—it's hard to stay away!), try setting boundaries. I started using app timers to limit how much I scroll, and it's made a huge difference. I realized I was spending more time comparing myself

to strangers than enjoying my own life. That's when I knew something had to change.

3. **Focus on What Brings You Joy**: Instead of getting caught up in the scroll, redirect your energy. One thing I started doing was making a nightly to-do list. It might sound small, but having simple tasks—like reading a chapter of a book or trying a new recipe—helped me stay grounded and present. Those moments of joy are worth so much more than the fleeting satisfaction of a "like" on social media.

THE TRUTH BEHIND SOCIAL MEDIA'S "PERFECT LIFE"

We've all been there—scrolling through Instagram or Facebook, admiring someone's luxury vacation, romantic gestures, or flawless selfies, and feeling a pang of comparison. Why doesn't my life look like that? Why can't I have it all together like they do? I've felt it too, more times than I'd like to admit. But here's what I've learned: social media is a highlight reel, not the full story. Behind every "perfect" post is a reality we don't see—the stressful arguments before the picture-perfect family photo, the endless takes to capture that glowing selfie, or the chaos that unfolded before the seemingly serene vacation shot. Life is messy, unpredictable, and beautifully imperfect for everyone, no matter how polished their posts appear.

Once I realized this, it was freeing. I stopped comparing my real, unfiltered life to someone else's curated feed. Instead, I shifted my focus inward, recognizing that true beauty and happiness come from embracing who we are, not from chasing likes or striving for unrealistic ideals. Real beauty is found in kindness, strength, and authenticity—qualities that can't be filtered or faked. So, the next time you feel tempted to compare, remind yourself: your worth isn't measured by someone else's highlight reel. It's found in the unique, imperfect, and extraordinary story that is yours alone. Let's stop scrolling and start living.

WAYS TO BOOST YOUR SELF-CONFIDENCE

1. **Unfollow Toxic Influences:** If someone's posts on Facebook, Instagram, or Snapchat make you feel inadequate, it's time to hit "unfollow." It's liberating to clear your feed of content that doesn't uplift or inspire you.
2. **Follow Body-Positive Accounts:** Surround yourself with people and accounts that promote diversity and positivity. Seek out influencers who champion self-love and showcase beauty in all forms— real, unfiltered, and unique.
3. **Set Goals Focused on Personal Growth:** Shift your focus from appearance to growth. Instead of fixating on your body, set realistic goals that build your confidence. Maybe it's learning a new skill, improving your health in meaningful ways (like committing to exercise or better nutrition), or dedicating time to your hobbies and passions.
4. **Dress to Empower Yourself:** What you wear can impact how you feel. Choose clothes that make you feel confident and comfortable, and don't be afraid to experiment with styles that express who you are.
5. **Limit Your Social Media Exposure:** Try setting strict time limits on your Facebook, Instagram, and Snapchat use. You can even schedule "offline" days to give your mind a break from the constant barrage of images and comparison.
6. **Cultivate Gratitude:** Gratitude is a powerful antidote to self-doubt. Each day, write down three things you're grateful for, whether they're big or small. This simple habit helps you focus on the positives in your life rather than on what you think you're missing.
7. **Find Joy in Real Connections:** Spend time with people who make you feel loved, supported, and appreciated. These real-life connections will do more

for your confidence than any amount of likes or comments ever could.

THE REAL MEANING OF BEAUTY: LOOKING BEYOND THE MIRROR

True beauty isn't just about what you see in the mirror; it's about how you move through the world with grace, the kindness you extend to others, and the love you nurture for yourself. It's found in the way you embrace your imperfections and celebrate your uniqueness. When you shift your focus from external appearances to your character and values, you unlock a level of confidence that no trend or standard can take away.

Beauty isn't about meeting societal expectations or chasing fleeting trends—it's about living authentically, in a way that honors who you truly are. When you embrace your natural self, your inner glow becomes undeniable. No filter, AI enhancement, or cosmetic procedure could ever replicate the radiance that comes from being unapologetically you.

IN SUMMARY – REFLECT AND RECLAIM YOUR CONFIDENCE

Confidence is the most radiant quality you can possess, and it comes from nurturing your mind, body, and soul—not from following trends or chasing unattainable ideals. True beauty lies in owning your uniqueness, embracing your imperfections, and allowing your inner strength to shine.

Social media—whether it's **Facebook, Instagram, TikTok, or Snapchat**—doesn't have to dictate how you see yourself. Instead of letting curated images and fleeting trends shape your worth, take back control. Pause for a moment and ask yourself: **Which app do I reach for most often? How does it make me feel? Could I spend less time scrolling and more time doing something meaningful?** Imagine using that time to learn a new skill, reignite an old passion, or simply connect with the people who truly matter to you.

Your time, energy, and self-worth are far too valuable to waste on comparisons. Let today be the day you choose to redefine beauty on your terms—to find joy in your reflection, in your growth, and in the life you're creating. Because when you prioritize what truly matters, you'll discover that your most beautiful self is already within you, waiting to shine.

CHAPTER 3
THE SOUNDTRACK OF YOUR LIFE
EMBRACING MUSIC THERAPY FOR BALANCE AND JOY

DISCOVERING MUSIC THERAPY AS A TOOL FOR BALANCE

During my journey to earn my advanced holistic nurse certification, I stumbled upon music therapy. Until then, I hadn't realized how powerful music could be as a form of therapy. It wasn't just about listening to my favorite tunes—it was about tuning in to sounds that could calm the mind, lift the spirit, and help me focus. I learned that music therapy wasn't about having a perfect playlist; it was about using music intentionally as a tool for mental and emotional well-being. In this chapter, I'll share how music therapy became a resource for me and how it can help you navigate life's stresses and find balance.

SECTION 1: WHAT IS MUSIC THERAPY? YOUR KEY TO EMOTIONAL WELLNESS

Music therapy is an intentional approach to using music to enhance mental and emotional health. It's about choosing sounds, rhythms, and melodies that help us release stress, connect with our emotions, and feel more grounded. Music therapists use these elements to support people in managing anxiety, improving focus, and finding a sense of peace.

Even if you're not working with a music therapist, you can still harness the benefits of music therapy by building mindful listening habits and creating playlists to suit your needs.

SECTION 2: THE SCIENCE OF SOUND: WHY MUSIC WORKS WONDERS FOR YOUR MIND

Music has always held a special place in my heart. Growing up, I loved to sing—it was my escape, my comfort, and my joy. Back then, life was simple. We didn't have electronics or endless toys to entertain us. What we did have was the radio, and it felt like magic. My siblings and I would gather around, listening to our favorite tunes, singing along, and letting the melodies transport us. During moments of stress or loneliness, I would hum a song or belt out a tune, and somehow, the world seemed brighter.

Now, as an adult, I understand why music had such a profound effect. When we listen to music, it sparks activity in different parts of the brain. It releases **dopamine**, the "feel-good" neurotransmitter, along with **endorphins**, which help ease tension and lift our spirits. While most **serotonin**—another key player in mood regulation—is produced in the gut, music helps stimulate dopamine and endorphin release in the brain, stabilizing mood, reducing stress, and creating a sense of calm.

For women, music therapy resonates deeply because it connects us to our emotions in such a unique way. It allows us to express, feel, and even release pent-up feelings in a safe and nurturing space. Whether it's a favorite song from childhood, a powerful anthem, or a soft instrumental piece, music gives us the opportunity to find comfort and strength in its embrace—just as it did for me all those years ago, sitting by the radio and feeling the world's troubles fade away.

SECTION 3: MUSIC FOR HEALING: TRANSFORMING ANXIETY AND FEAR INTO CALM AND STRENGTH

I'll never forget the overwhelming anxiety I felt before my C-section. The anticipation, the uncertainty—it all felt like too much. In those moments, I turned to music. I chose calming, relaxing melodies, letting the gentle notes carry my mind to a more peaceful place. It didn't make the situation disappear, but it gave me something soothing to focus on, grounding me when my thoughts were spiraling.

Working as a nurse, I've seen firsthand how music can transform a tense atmosphere. In hospitals and surgery centers, turning on soft, soothing background music in waiting rooms or pre-surgery areas can make a world of difference. I've watched patients take deeper breaths, their shoulders relax, and a sense of calm settle over them as the music worked its quiet magic.

How Music Can Reduce Anxiety in Clinical Settings

- The power of music to lower anxiety is undeniable. It slows the heart rate, lowers **cortisol** (the body's stress hormone), and creates an environment where relaxation feels possible. It's why so many hospitals use it intentionally—to make an inherently stressful setting feel just a little more manageable.
- If you're ever facing an anxious moment—whether it's a big meeting, a tough conversation, or even just a particularly overwhelming day—try creating your own "calm zone." Put on soothing instrumental tracks or nature-inspired sounds and let them ease your mind.

Music therapy is such a simple yet powerful tool. It's not just about enjoying a good tune; it's about intentionally using music to shift your mindset, soothe your nerves, and help you find peace, even in the most challenging moments.

SECTION 4: USING MUSIC INTENTIONALLY: HOW TO BUILD A PLAYLIST FOR YOUR SOUL

Music has always been my companion during life's most stressful or emotional moments. I vividly recall the night before my wedding—a mix of excitement and nerves left my mind racing. To calm myself, I played some gentle acoustic tunes, and as the music filled the room, my heart began to steady. It didn't erase the jitters entirely, but it gave me the clarity and calm I needed to focus on the joy of the moment.

Another time was during my nursing board exam preparation. The pressure to succeed felt immense, and the thought of failure loomed large. I would turn to uplifting playlists that not only kept me motivated but also brought a sense of comfort amidst the grind. Music became my steadying force, helping me stay grounded and focused.

As a nurse, I've witnessed the profound ways music can touch lives, even in the most challenging moments. I recall patients who had just received life-altering diagnoses, their faces etched with fear and uncertainty. In these moments, when words often fell short, I noticed how a gentle melody could create a space of calm. For patients grappling with the weight of a terminal illness, music became more than background noise—it became a source of solace, offering a momentary escape from the overwhelming reality. I've seen families in hospital rooms, gathered around a loved one, find comfort in a shared song that reminded them of better times. Music, in those moments, acted as a bridge, connecting them to the hope and strength they didn't realize they had. It's a universal balm—a quiet, powerful way to soothe not just the body, but the soul, even when the path ahead feels uncertain.

Intentional use of music is all about choosing sounds with a purpose—whether that's to calm your mind, energize your body, or bring clarity to your thoughts. For instance, after a tough day, gentle piano music can feel like a warm hug, helping you wind down and reset. On the flip side, an upbeat rhythm can snap you out of an energy slump, giving you that little boost to finish your day strong.

Harnessing the Power of Music for Relaxation

When life feels overwhelming, music can be a lifeline. The secret? Matching the tempo of the music to your mood. A tempo of 60–80 beats per minute (BPM) is particularly effective because it mirrors your resting heart rate, encouraging your body and mind to naturally relax. Here's how you can make it work for you:

Why 60–80 BPM Works

This tempo creates a calming effect by syncing with your body's natural rhythm. It's like a gentle nudge telling your heart and mind, "Slow down, it's time to unwind." Whether you're stressed, anxious, or simply need to refocus, this range of BPM helps you center yourself and breathe more deeply.

How to Find 60–80 BPM Music

1. **Tap Along to the Beat**
   - Count the beats in 15 seconds and multiply by 4 to estimate the BPM. It's a quick and easy way to find songs that match the tempo you need.
2. **Use Apps for Precision**
   - Apps like BPM Detector can instantly identify the tempo of your favorite tracks. It's a great way to build a playlist of relaxing music.
3. **Search Curated Playlists**
   - Platforms like **Spotify**, **YouTube**, and **Apple Music** have playlists specifically labeled by BPM.

Simply search terms like "Relaxing Music 60 BPM" or "Calm Playlist 70 BPM" to discover tracks designed for relaxation.

4. **Opt for Pre-Made Mindfulness Tracks**
    o Many mindfulness and relaxation tracks are intentionally composed at 60–80 BPM. Look for music tagged with BPM details in the titles or descriptions, especially in genres like instrumental, classical, or ambient music.

Making It Work for You

Imagine this: You've had a tough day, and your mind is racing. You pop in your earbuds, find a 60 BPM playlist, and within minutes, the slow rhythm starts syncing with your body. You feel your breath ease and your shoulders drop. That's the magic of finding the right tempo—your internal chaos starts to settle.

By incorporating these simple techniques, you can make music your go-to tool for relaxation, helping you reset and recharge, one beat at a time. So, the next time life feels a little too loud, let the soothing rhythm of 60–80 BPM music guide you back to calm.

Create Purposeful Playlists

Music is more than just background noise—it's a powerful tool to shape your mood and energy. By creating playlists tailored to your emotions or activities, you can use music as a purposeful ally in your daily life.

*   **For Calm**: Fill your playlist with soothing instrumental tracks, ambient sounds, or soft classical music. It is perfect for unwinding after a hectic day or preparing for a peaceful night's sleep.
*   **For Focus**: Choose classical pieces or lo-fi beats to create a productive atmosphere for work, study, or creative endeavors.

- **For Energy**: Energizing pop hits, rhythmic Latin beats, or high-tempo anthems can give you the boost you need for a workout, cleaning spree, or long drive.

Making Music a Daily Ritual: Finding Harmony in Everyday Moments

Incorporate music into your daily routines to create moments of joy, balance, and calm:

- **Morning Motivation**: Start your day with upbeat tracks that energize you for the challenges ahead.
- **Midday Recharge**: Use calming sounds or ambient melodies during lunch to refocus and recharge.
- **Evening Wind-Down**: Close your day with gentle tunes to help your mind and body relax before bedtime.

When in Doubt, Search Smart

Not sure where to start? Platforms like YouTube, Spotify, and Apple Music have endless options. Try searching for terms like:

- "Relaxing background music"
- "Calm instrumental"
- "Focus music"
- "Energizing workout songs"

These curated playlists are ready to meet your specific needs, whether you're seeking stillness or a spark of energy.

MUSIC: YOUR COMPANION FOR LIFE

Using Music in Everyday Moments for a Calm State of Mind

Life can feel overwhelming at times, but music has a way of cutting through the chaos. To keep anxiety at bay, try setting aside small, intentional music breaks throughout your day. Think of it as a mini-retreat: five minutes of peaceful melodies to start your morning, a calming tune during your work break, or gentle music in the evening to help you wind down. It's amazing how just a few minutes of the right music can reset your mind and make everything feel a little more manageable.

Making Music Therapy a Personal Practice

Music therapy doesn't have to be complicated. It's about finding what works for you and weaving it into your daily life. Here are some practical and engaging ways to make music a part of your personal wellness routine:

1. Create Your Personal "Mood-Boosting" Playlist

- Imagine having a playlist that's like a toolkit for your emotions—relaxation, motivation, joy, calm. Building this kind of playlist can be a game-changer.
- Apps like Spotify or Apple Music make it easy. Search for playlists with names like "Calming Vibes," "Mood Boosters," or "Feel-Good Hits." Save your favorites, so they're always ready when you need them.
- **Pro Tip**: Apps like **Calm** and **Headspace** offer curated playlists designed for mental wellness, such as "Relaxing Melodies" or "Energy Boost" These are perfect if you need something quick and effective.

2. Music Therapy for Driving: Stay Focused and Engaged on the Road

Driving often feels like a chore, but it can also be an ideal time for intentional music therapy. Upbeat tunes with steady rhythms can help you stay alert and focused. Think pop anthems, energetic rock, or even a little dance music to keep your spirits high.

- **Action Tip**: Build a driving playlist with your favorite energizing songs. Platforms like Spotify or YouTube have ready-made "Driving Playlists" to save you time.
- Songs with steady beats in the range of 90–120 BPM (beats per minute) are particularly great for keeping your focus sharp without feeling overstimulated.

3. Understanding the Magic of a Steady Beat

What is a steady beat? It's the musical equivalent of a heartbeat —a rhythm that stays consistent throughout the song.

- **Why It Helps**: Songs with steady beats between 90–120 BPM sync naturally with your energy, keeping you focused and alert without adding stress.
- **How to Find Steady Beat Music**:
    - Use platforms like Spotify or Apple Music to search for playlists labeled with BPM ranges, such as "90 BPM playlist" or "100 BPM focus music."
    - Besides BPM Detector, as mentioned earlier, you can use apps like **Song BPM** or **BPM Counter** to identify the BPM of your favorite songs and build a custom playlist.
    - Explore genres like pop, rock, or lo-fi for songs with naturally steady rhythms.
    - YouTube also has endless options—just search for terms like "steady beat playlist" or "90 BPM driving music."

4. Leveraging YouTube and Music Apps for Specific Needs

YouTube is a treasure trove of mood-based music. Channels like **Relaxing White Noise** and **Meditation Relax Music** cater to specific needs, offering everything from stress relief to focus and motivation.

- **Simple Search Tips**: Use keywords like "morning motivation," "focus music," or "stress relief music" to find curated tracks that fit your moment.
- **Create a "Music Therapy" Playlist**: Save your favorite YouTube videos to a playlist titled "Music Therapy." This way, you'll have an easy-to-access collection ready to lift your mood, help you focus, or bring calm whenever you need it.

Music as Your Daily Companion

Music isn't just for entertainment—it's a reliable partner in navigating life's ups and downs. Whether it's calming your nerves before a big presentation, turning a frustrating commute into a karaoke session, or helping you center yourself during a tough day, music is always there.

As women juggling countless roles—caregiver, professional, friend, partner—it's easy to feel stretched thin. But music is like a little secret weapon, a simple way to nurture your well-being in moments that might otherwise feel overwhelming.

"When words fail, music speaks." Let it speak to you in the small, quiet spaces of your day, helping you find balance, strength, and joy. Whether it's through a carefully curated playlist or a single soothing melody, let music remind you that every day is an opportunity to create harmony—inside and out.

5. Making Music Therapy Flexible and Family-Friendly

One of the best things about music therapy is its adaptability—it works for you, your schedule, and even your family. Use it "as needed" for a quick mood boost or weave it into your daily routine. Start your morning with uplifting beats, play soothing tunes before bed, or use calming melodies to ease into a busy workday. If time is tight, even five-minute sessions can make a big impact—consistency is key.

But music therapy doesn't have to be a solo experience. It's a wonderful way to bring peace and connection into your family life. Play calming music during dinner for a serene atmosphere, or pump up the energy with cheerful tunes on weekend mornings. This shared experience can be a positive bonding tool and help everyone de-stress.

- **Family Tip**: Create a "happy playlist" together. Let everyone contribute their favorite songs, whether for a lively start to the day or a relaxing bedtime routine.

6. Recommended Playlists and Channels

Finding the right music can feel overwhelming, but there are plenty of curated playlists and channels to simplify the process. Apps like **Calm** and **Headspace**, as mentioned earlier, specialize in music for focus, stress relief, and sleep. Platforms like **Spotify** and **YouTube** also offer ready-to-go options for any mood. Here are some ideas to explore:

- **Spotify**: "Chill Vibes," "Peaceful Piano," "Mood Booster"
- **YouTube Channels: Relaxing White Noise, Calm Whale, YellowBrickCinema**

Start with these suggestions and tailor your playlists as you discover what resonates most with you and your family.

SECTION 5: MAKING MUSIC THERAPY A ROUTINE FOR LASTING IMPACT

Music therapy works best when it becomes a natural part of your daily life, not just an occasional afterthought. Let's dive into how you can weave music into your routine effortlessly—and maybe even have a little fun along the way.

1. Set Intentional Music Moments

Let's face it: life is hectic, and carving out time for yourself can feel like a luxury. But music therapy doesn't have to take hours; even five minutes can work wonders.

- Self-Care Sundays: Picture this—your favorite face mask, a warm cup of tea, and a playlist of calming acoustic songs in the background. Bliss, right?
- Power Mornings: If you're juggling work, kids, and the occasional existential crisis, start your day with upbeat, empowering tunes. It's like coffee for your soul.
- Evening Wind-Down: After a day of managing everyone else's needs, play soft piano music during your bedtime routine. It's your time to reset and recharge.

2. Pair Music with Movement

Why not make your daily activities a little more enjoyable? Music can turn even the most mundane tasks into something bearable—maybe even fun.

- Gentle yoga or stretching with soothing sounds can double as "you time."
- Turn chore time into a mini dance party. Folding laundry is less boring when Beyoncé is reminding you, "Who runs the world? (Hint: it's you).
- For workouts, find a playlist with steady beats to keep you motivated—even when that last squat feels impossible.

- **New Tip:** If your energy dips during your monthly cycle, have playlists ready to match your mood: calming on tough days and energizing when you're ready to conquer the world again.

3. Music as a Confidence Booster

We all have those moments—before a big presentation, a first date, or even just a daunting Monday morning. Music can be your secret weapon.

- Play your "power song" to channel your inner superstar. (Mine's Roar by Katy Perry—what's yours?)
- Create a playlist of songs by women who inspire strength and resilience. Share it with your besties for an instant mood lift.
- **Pro Tip:** Keep that playlist handy. Some days, you just need an anthem to remind you how amazing you are.

4. Keep Playlists Fresh

Ever realize you've been listening to the same playlist for months? Guilty. It's time to shake things up.

- Rotate your playlists regularly. Add songs from different cultures—African beats, Latin rhythms, or Indian sitar music can give your routine a fresh vibe.
- Try apps like Endel, which create soundscapes based on your mood and environment. It's like a personal DJ who actually understands you.
- **Quick Fix:** Challenge yourself to find one new song each week. It's a small change that can completely transform your listening experience.

5. Reconnect with Yourself Through Music

Life's demands can sometimes make you feel like you've lost

touch with who you are. Music therapy is a beautiful way to reconnect.

- Play songs that remind you of your younger, carefree self. (Spice Girls fans, where are you at?)
- Curate a playlist that encourages reflection and dreaming. Think of it as your personal soundtrack for self-discovery.
- **Personal Tip:** I've found that revisiting nostalgic songs not only lifts my mood but also reminds me of how far I've come. Try it—you'll be surprised by the memories and emotions that surface.

6. Make It a Family Affair

Music isn't just for you; it's a great way to bond with loved ones.

- Start the weekend with a family dance-off in the living room. (Bonus: It counts as cardio.)
- Play calming melodies during dinner to create a relaxing atmosphere.
- Build a collaborative playlist where everyone adds their favorite tracks. It's a fun way to connect and discover new music together.
- **Fun Idea:** Let your kids pick a song to start each morning. You'll either laugh or cringe—but either way, it's a memory in the making.

Fresh Ideas to Make It Unique

- DIY Sound Therapy: Create calming sounds at home with wind chimes or gentle humming. Who says you can't be your own music therapist?
- Women-Centric Playlists: Build a playlist of empowering songs by female artists. Need a pick-me-up? Beyoncé, Adele, or Lizzo are just a few clicks away.

With these tips, music therapy becomes more than just background noise—it's your ally in finding calm, focus, and joy. Let music be the little nudge that helps you navigate life's chaos with grace and confidence.

CONCLUSION: EMBRACE THE HARMONY OF MUSIC THERAPY

Music isn't just sound—it's a divine gift, a sanctuary, and a bridge to moments of peace and joy that can feel out of reach in the chaos of daily life. It's something we often listen to without a second thought, taking for granted the profound ways it can heal and uplift us. But when we pause and reflect, we can truly thank God for the creation of music—a universal language that connects our minds and souls in extraordinary ways.

The beauty of music therapy lies in its simplicity. You don't need fancy equipment or hours of free time—just a song that resonates with you, a few quiet moments, and a willingness to let it work its magic. Think about the last time music truly moved you. Maybe it was a melody that brought tears of release when life felt heavy, or a beat that lifted your spirits when you were at your lowest. Those moments aren't coincidences—they're proof of music's incredible ability to touch the deepest parts of us.

By using music intentionally, with purpose and mindfulness, you can unlock its full benefits for your mind and soul. It's a tool to reset, recharge, and reconnect—not just with yourself, but with those around you. Play a calming tune during family time, sing along with your kids in the car, or share a playlist with a friend who's struggling. Music has the power to create harmony not just in our hearts but in our relationships, too.

I've seen music bring calm to patients facing daunting diagnoses, and I've felt its power myself in moments of fear and uncertainty. It's not just therapy—it's an act of gratitude and self-love. So, give yourself permission to pause, press play, and let music be the companion that lifts you up and carries you forward.

You don't have to chase perfection to find balance. You already have the tools within you, and music is one of the simplest, yet most profound, ways to unlock that inner harmony. Let's not take this gift for granted any longer—use it with intention, as a way to heal, grow, and thrive. Turn up the volume on your well-being—one note at a time.

CHAPTER 4
THE MIND-BEAUTY CONNECTION
THE HIDDEN POWER OF YOUR THOUGHTS TO TRANSFORM YOUR SKIN AND CONFIDENCE

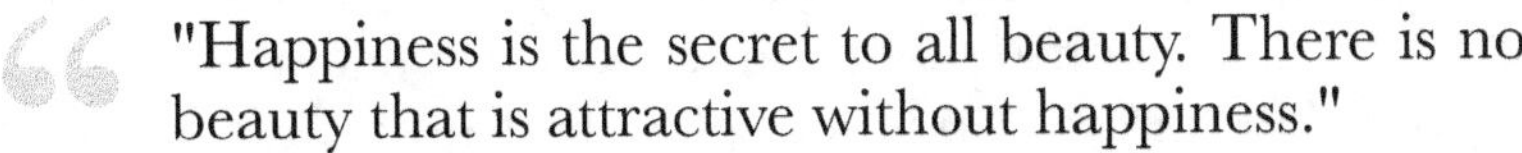

"Happiness is the secret to all beauty. There is no beauty that is attractive without happiness."

— Christian Dior

Let's pause for a moment. Can you think of the last time you had a bad day? Picture it: you felt drained, your posture slumped, eye contact became scarce, and every word seemed to come out in a monotone. Perhaps there were sighs that punctuated the silence, as if your whole body was broadcasting your inner struggles. Now, contrast that with a great day—one where you felt unstoppable. You were smiling, standing tall, your voice carried energy, and your confidence was palpable. Here's the truth: how you feel inside doesn't just stay there—it shows on the outside.

WHEN YOUR MOOD IMPACTS YOUR APPEARANCE

It's no secret that a bad mood doesn't just affect your mental state—it seeps into how you look and act. Maybe you notice your skin looking dull, new breakouts appearing, or even dark circles creeping under your eyes. Your body language follows suit, with slouched shoulders and a lack of enthusiasm in your movements.

But it doesn't stop there. When your mental health takes a hit, self-care often becomes a casualty. Think about it—how often do bad days lead to skipping your skincare routine, reaching for junk food instead of something nourishing, or deciding to skip your workout entirely? Over time, this neglect adds up. The cycle is vicious: you feel low, you stop taking care of yourself, and then your physical appearance reflects that neglect, reinforcing those feelings of inadequacy.

Here's the empowering part: breaking this cycle starts with understanding the connection between your mind and your beauty. When you nurture your inner self, it reflects outwardly, giving you that natural, confident glow that no beauty product can replicate. Together, we'll explore how cultivating mental wellness can elevate your physical presence, creating a harmony that radiates from the inside out.

THE LINK BETWEEN DEPRESSION AND OUTER BEAUTY

We've all experienced days when we look in the mirror and feel less than our best. But what happens when a low mood becomes more than just a fleeting feeling—when it takes root and clouds not only our mind but also the way we see ourselves? That's the insidious nature of depression: it doesn't just affect how we feel; it changes how we perceive ourselves, often dimming the light of our inner and outer beauty.

When depression settles in, even the simplest acts of self-care—like brushing your hair, applying a touch of lipstick, or picking out an outfit that makes you feel confident—can feel overwhelming. A routine shower might feel like climbing a mountain. The joy we once found in pampering ourselves disappears, replaced by a sense of apathy or exhaustion.

And then there's the mind's cruel trick: depression distorts our self-image. We start comparing ourselves to others, convinced we don't measure up. It's as if we're looking at our reflection through a foggy mirror, one that only highlights flaws and drowns out any sense of worthiness or beauty. These negative thought spirals isolate us further, creating a cycle that feels impossible to break.

But here's the truth: you are not alone, and depression does not define you. With the right tools and support, you can reclaim not just your mental well-being but also the confidence and joy that come from embracing your unique beauty.

TACKLING DEPRESSION: PRACTICAL STEPS TO RECLAIM YOURSELF

If depression has cast its shadow over your life—or the life of someone you love—know that healing is possible. Here are some steps to help navigate this journey back to self-love and well-being:

Reach Out for Professional Help.

- Depression isn't a battle you have to fight alone. Mental health professionals, like therapists or counselors, are trained to guide you through this journey. Techniques like cognitive-behavioral therapy (CBT) can help reshape those distorted thoughts, offering tools to build resilience and a brighter outlook.

Open Up to Your Circle

- Depression often whispers lies that we're a burden or that no one understands. But opening up to a trusted friend or family member can shatter that illusion. Sharing your feelings with someone who truly cares can lighten the emotional load and remind you that support is always within reach.

Explore Medical Treatment If Needed

- Sometimes, the chemical imbalances linked to depression require medical intervention. If you feel comfortable, talk to your doctor about the possibility of medication. Remember, there's no shame in seeking help. Antidepressants aren't a weakness—they're a tool, like glasses for the mind, to help you see life more clearly again.

Focus on Small, Daily Wins

- When depression makes everything feel impossible, start small. Pick one manageable task each day—a five-minute skincare routine, a walk around the block, or even just making your bed. These small victories aren't just actions; they're proof that you're moving forward, one step at a time.

A PERSONAL NOTE: REDISCOVERING JOY IN THE LITTLE THINGS

I've seen this journey up close, not only in my patients but in my own moments of struggle. I remember a patient who came to me feeling utterly lost. Her depression had taken away her motivation to care for herself, and her once-radiant confidence seemed like a distant memory. Together, we worked on simple, actionable steps—she started with a short morning routine, just washing her face and putting on her favorite lotion. Over time, those small habits snowballed into bigger changes, reigniting her sense of self.

The thing about depression is that it's persistent, but so is hope. Each little step—no matter how small—carries you closer to rediscovering the vibrant, beautiful person you are. Remember, beauty isn't about perfection; it's about resilience.

So, if you're reading this and feeling stuck, know this: you are worth the effort. Start with a small act of kindness for yourself today. Tomorrow, take another. And the next day, another still. Slowly but surely, you'll find your way back to the person you've always been—strong, radiant, and beautifully you.

Focus on Daily Habits: Developing consistent daily routines —no matter how small—can help combat feelings of overwhelm and inertia. Whether it's a five-minute skincare routine, making your bed, or walking outside for fresh air, these simple actions can build momentum and lift your spirits over time.

Remember, recovery takes time, but with the right combination of support—professional help, social connection, and self-care —you can begin to feel like yourself again.

HOW STRESS AFFECTS OUR BEAUTY

Stress doesn't just weigh on your mind—it leaves its mark on your skin, hair, and overall appearance. Ever noticed that after a tough week, you seem to wake up with more breakouts, dull skin, or even a few extra fine lines? That's stress working its behind-the-scenes magic—and not in a good way.

When we're stressed, our body pumps out cortisol, also known as the "stress hormone." While cortisol is helpful for quick bursts of energy during emergencies (like escaping a near-accident), chronic stress means consistently high cortisol levels, which can disrupt almost every system in your body—including the ones responsible for keeping you glowing.

Let's break it down:

Wrinkles and Fine Lines

- Cortisol breaks down collagen, the protein that keeps your skin firm and elastic. Without collagen, your skin starts to lose its bounce, and wrinkles and sagging can creep in earlier than you'd like. It's as if stress is sending your skin an unwanted "time travel" invitation

—straight to the future of premature aging.

Breakouts and Blemishes

- Feeling stressed and noticing more acne? You're not imagining things. Stress ramps up oil production, clogging your pores and leading to unwelcome breakouts. Whether it's a full-blown flare-up or just a few stubborn blemishes, stress has a knack for showing up on your face.

Hair Loss and Thinning

- Ever run your fingers through your hair during a stressful time and feel like more strands are falling out? Stress can cause your body to hit the pause button on "non-essential" functions like hair growth, leading to thinning or shedding over time. This condition, called telogen effluvium, might not be permanent, but it's certainly unwelcome.

TRANSITION: FROM AWARENESS TO ACTION

Understanding how stress affects your beauty is only half the battle. The good news is that by managing stress, you're not just protecting your inner well-being—you're giving your outer beauty a much-needed boost, too. After all, the best beauty regimen starts from within.

Here are a few stress-management techniques to consider as you reclaim your natural glow:

- **Breathing Exercises:** A few deep breaths can help calm your nervous system and lower cortisol levels in minutes.
- **Prioritize Sleep:** Rest is your body's time to heal and repair. Protect your beauty sleep—it's called that

for a reason!

- **Hydrate and Nourish:** Stress can dehydrate your skin, so drink plenty of water and eat nutrient-rich foods that support your body and beauty.
- **Movement and Mindfulness:** A quick walk or a few moments of meditation can do wonders for both your mood and your skin.

Stress doesn't have to dictate how you feel—or how you look. By taking small steps to manage it, you're not only building resilience but also giving yourself the best gift: a mind and body that radiate calm, confidence, and beauty.

EXERCISE: A BOOST FOR BOTH BEAUTY AND MIND

We all know exercise is great for staying fit, but it's also a beauty secret that works from the inside out. When you move, your body releases endorphins, those feel-good hormones that instantly lift your mood and help fight anxiety and depression. Beyond the mental boost, regular movement improves circulation, delivering more oxygen and nutrients to your skin for that natural, healthy glow.

And here's the bonus: when paired with mindful breathing —like in yoga or stretching—exercise activates the body's natural relaxation system, the parasympathetic nervous system, which lowers cortisol levels and reduces the harmful effects of stress. Think of it as your beauty and mood enhancer rolled into one!

CONCLUSION: EMPOWERING YOUR BEAUTY THROUGH THE MIND-BODY CONNECTION

Your beauty isn't just skin deep—it's a reflection of the harmony between your mind and body. How you feel inside profoundly impacts how you look outside. Confidence and contentment radiate as improved posture, brighter eyes, and a natural glow—traits that no makeup can replicate. On the other hand, stress, anxiety, and neglect can show up as dull skin, tension lines, or low energy.

The good news is that you hold the power to cultivate this positive mind-beauty connection. By prioritizing mental wellness, practicing self-compassion, and nurturing your inner beauty, you can transform how you feel and look. This isn't about perfection—it's about embracing your authentic self and making choices that align with your well-being.

Every small, intentional step—whether taking a deep breath, practicing gratitude, or walking in nature—builds the foundation for lasting beauty and wellness. Your glow comes not just from how you care for your appearance but from the love and kindness you show to yourself and others.

You deserve to feel beautiful, confident, and strong—not just in fleeting moments but every day. Choose to honor your mind and body, and the world will see the light you shine.

CHAPTER 5
ELEVATE YOUR LIFE
THE JOURNEY OF HOLISTIC SELF-CARE AND EMPOWERMENT

Self-care, much like self-development, isn't a straight path. It's a journey of ebbs and flows, filled with moments of growth and times of struggle. Some days, caring for yourself feels like second nature; other days, it feels like an uphill climb. And that's okay. These challenges are not setbacks—they're stepping stones. True self-care isn't about achieving perfection; it's about showing up for yourself, embracing the process, and finding peace in simply being present with who you are.

As Dr. Masaru Emoto beautifully reminds us:

> "If you feel lost, disappointed, hesitant, or weak, return to yourself—to who you are, here and now. And when you get there, you will discover yourself, like a lotus flower in full bloom, even in a muddy pond: beautiful and strong."

When we take the time to reconnect with ourselves—our inner beauty, strength, and purpose—we bloom. Like the lotus flower rising from the mud, we emerge stronger, more radiant, and more grounded in our true selves.

This journey of self-care and self-discovery is an invitation to live fully in the present, to let go of external pressures, and to embrace the beauty that already exists within you. No matter the challenges or the muddy waters, you are capable of blooming into the fullest, most beautiful version of yourself.

THE POWER OF HOLISTIC SELF-CARE

Holistic self-care goes beyond the surface—it's more than running, skincare routines, or weight management. It's an intentional practice that nurtures your mind, body, and spirit in harmony, allowing you to connect with your true self. When self-care becomes just another item on a to-do list, its deeper purpose gets lost. But when approached holistically, it transforms into a journey of growth, healing, and self-discovery.

True self-care starts from within. It's about making choices from a place of stillness and connection—becoming aware of your senses, your possibilities, and even your higher consciousness. This isn't just about ticking boxes for today's routines; it's about embracing a lifelong process of learning, evolving, and becoming more aligned with who you truly are.

Let's be honest—few of us were ever taught to pause and check in with how we're feeling inside. We rarely stop to understand our own experiences or what it means to be fully present. Yet this is where real growth begins. By learning to regulate your attention and set your intention, you're planting the seeds for profound personal development. Small practices, like taking moments for reflection, listening to your inner voice, or simply being present, create the foundation for deeper self-care that nourishes every part of your being.

Every journey needs preparation, and self-care is no different. Start by asking yourself: Why am I doing this? What do I need right now? When you clarify your purpose, it becomes easier to make choices that align with your true needs. Think of it like planning a trip: you set your destination, map out the route, and pack only what serves you. Along the way, you assess your progress, adjust your plans, and remind yourself why you started.

Holistic self-care isn't about rushing through checklists or chasing perfection. It's about showing up for yourself in a way that feels meaningful and intentional. Take a few deep breaths, focus on what you truly need, and give yourself permission to slow down. This journey isn't a race—it's a lifelong commitment to honoring and caring for the most important relationship you'll ever have: the one with yourself.

So start small. Take one intentional step today—whether it's a quiet moment to reflect, a walk outside to reconnect with nature, or simply acknowledging your feelings without judgment. With every mindful choice, you're creating space for growth, peace, and a deeper connection to your inner self.

NURTURING YOURSELF: THE PATH TO CONFIDENCE AND BALANCE

Holistic self-care isn't just about pampering yourself—it's about creating a life where you feel empowered, confident, and aligned with your true self. When you invest time in caring for your mind, body, and soul, you're not only boosting your confidence but also laying the foundation for a more balanced and fulfilling life. Let's explore practical ways to prioritize self-care and unlock the confidence within you.

1. Move Your Body, Elevate Your Mood

Exercise isn't just about physical fitness—it's a powerful tool to uplift your mental state. When you move, your body releases endorphins, those magical "feel-good" chemicals that reduce stress and spark joy. Whether it's yoga, a brisk walk, or a dance party in your living room, moving your body regularly keeps your energy high and your confidence soaring.

- **Tip:** Pair exercise with mindful breathing to engage your body's relaxation system. Even 10 minutes of stretching can create a sense of calm and clarity.

2. Build Real Connections

In a world of virtual interactions, genuine connections can feel rare, but they're essential for emotional well-being. Spending time with friends or family, sharing your thoughts, or simply laughing together releases oxytocin, the "bonding hormone," which naturally lowers stress and boosts happiness.

- **Action Step:** Schedule regular catch-ups with loved ones or join a supportive community where you can share experiences and feel understood.

3. Prioritize Self-Care Rituals

Self-care doesn't have to be extravagant—it's about finding small, meaningful ways to nurture yourself daily. Whether it's journaling, soaking in a warm bath, or enjoying your morning coffee in silence, these moments of "me-time" remind you that you're worth the care and attention.

- **Pro Tip:** Create a simple self-care schedule. For example, dedicate Sunday evenings to a face mask and your favorite book or podcast.

4. Fuel Your Body, Fuel Your Confidence

Your diet plays a pivotal role in how you feel and look. Nourishing yourself with whole, vibrant foods not only boosts your physical energy but also supports a positive mindset. On the flip side, overly processed foods can drain your energy and cloud your emotions.

- **Easy Swap:** Replace sugary snacks with a handful of nuts or fresh fruit. Small changes add up, and your body will thank you.

5. Challenge Negative Self-Talk

We all have that inner critic who whispers doubts and comparisons. The key is not to silence it but to challenge it. When a negative thought arises, ask yourself, "Is this true?" More often than not, it's not.

- **Practice:** Replace "I'm not good enough" with "I'm growing and learning every day." Over time, these affirmations can transform your self-perception.

6. Set Small Wins to Celebrate Big Gains

Confidence isn't built overnight—it's the result of small, consistent victories. Setting achievable goals and celebrating progress creates momentum and reinforces a sense of accomplishment.

- **Quick Idea:** Start with micro-goals like drinking an extra glass of water each day or organizing a single drawer. Every win, no matter how small, counts.

7. Laugh Often, Love Deeply

Laughter truly is the best medicine, and connecting with others brings joy and fulfillment. Sharing a joke, reminiscing with loved ones, or even watching a funny video can lift your spirits and remind you of the beauty in everyday life.

- **Lighthearted Challenge:** Spend 10 minutes a day doing something that makes you laugh—whether it's a sitcom, a funny meme, or a playful moment with your kids.

YOUR CONFIDENCE JOURNEY STARTS HERE

Self-care isn't a luxury—it's a necessity. By nurturing yourself, you're building the foundation for confidence that radiates from within. Remember, self-care and confidence are lifelong journeys, not destinations. Celebrate every step you take, and don't be afraid to stumble—it's all part of the process.

When you prioritize yourself, you're not just investing in your own well-being—you're creating a ripple effect of positivity for everyone around you. So, start small, stay consistent, and watch as your confidence grows, one intentional act of care at a time.

SHIFTING FROM EXTERNAL VALIDATION TO INNER CONFIDENCE

In today's fast-paced, social media-driven world, it's easy to find yourself chasing validation—whether it's the thrill of more likes on Instagram, compliments from others, or meeting society's ever-changing beauty standards. But here's the truth: lasting confidence doesn't come from what others see in you; it's rooted in how you see yourself.

Embracing Inner Beauty

The first step toward inner confidence is recognizing that beauty is more than skin-deep. Real beauty lies in your character, your resilience, and the way you treat others. When you shift your focus inward, you start to see yourself as a whole person—complete with strengths, quirks, and imperfections that make you uniquely you. This kind of self-acceptance creates a confidence that isn't easily shaken by external opinions or fleeting trends.

- **Reflection Exercise:** Take a moment to write down three qualities you love about yourself that have nothing to do with appearance. Keep this list where you can see it as a daily reminder of your inner beauty.

Redefining Self-Worth

Instead of measuring your worth by external factors, start connecting with the things that genuinely make you feel fulfilled. Maybe it's the satisfaction of helping a friend, the growth you experience through learning, or the peace you find in moments of stillness. These acts nourish your soul and remind you that your value isn't tied to how others perceive you.

- **Action Step:** Each day, do one thing that brings you joy or personal growth—whether it's journaling, practicing gratitude, or simply taking a walk in nature.

Letting Go of Unrealistic Standards

The media bombards us with images of perfection that are often unattainable, leaving us feeling like we're never "enough." But here's the secret: even those images are curated, filtered, and far from reality. Shifting your focus from achieving these impossible ideals to embracing your authentic self is where true confidence begins.

- **Lighthearted Tip:** When you catch yourself comparing, remind yourself that even supermodels don't wake up looking like their Instagram photos. Sometimes, we all need a laugh to shake off the pressure.

Building Confidence from Within

Cultivating inner confidence isn't about ignoring the world around you—it's about finding balance. When you prioritize inner peace and personal growth, you'll find that external validation matters less. Instead of seeking approval from others, you'll discover the freedom and joy of living authentically.

- **Remember:** Confidence is an inside job. When you stop chasing validation from others and start celebrating the amazing person you already are, you unlock a kind of beauty and strength that no trend or social media post can take away.

THE RHYTHM OF SELF-DEVELOPMENT: FINDING YOURSELF THROUGH LIFE'S UPS AND DOWNS

Self-development isn't a straight path; it's a rhythm—a dance between progress and setbacks, growth and reflection. You're invited to find yourself within this rhythm, to embrace the ups and downs as part of your unique journey. Challenges, like the storms we face in life, hold valuable lessons. They push us to stretch beyond our comfort zones and shape us into stronger, wiser, and more resilient versions of ourselves.

As we move toward a place of inner peace and acceptance, we begin to let go of the need to control every outcome. Instead of being attached to results, we can live fully in the moment, experiencing life with openness and curiosity. It's not about perfection; it's about presence—being with yourself as you are, and allowing growth to unfold naturally.

Reflective exercises can play a pivotal role in this process. Take time to ask yourself meaningful questions: What am I learning from this experience? How can I grow through this challenge? Journaling or meditating on these reflections can uncover insights that guide you toward becoming the best version of yourself. This intentional practice helps you connect with your deeper self, paving the way for authentic growth and self-awareness.

Remember, self-development is not about rushing to a finish line—it's about living the experience, embracing the lessons, and finding beauty in the process.

CONCLUSION: CELEBRATE THE POWER OF HOLISTIC SELF-CARE

Self-care is more than a series of tasks; it's an act of self-love, a declaration that you are worthy of time, effort, and nurturing. It's about planting seeds of intention, kindness, and growth in the rich soil of your being and watching as they bloom into the vibrant flowers of confidence, resilience, and inner peace. Every small act of care, every moment of reflection, and every step toward self-development is a testament to your commitment to yourself.

Through holistic self-care, you've embraced more than just routines; you've cultivated a life that values balance, inner beauty, and growth. From letting go of external validation to finding strength in reflection and connection, you've discovered the profound truth: your worth is not defined by anyone or anything but by the unique light that shines within you.

Celebrate yourself—the you who makes space for rest, joy, and growth. Celebrate the moments when you chose to move your body to release stress, to eat mindfully to nourish your soul, and to challenge negative thoughts with kindness. Celebrate the courage it takes to shift from seeking validation outside to finding confidence within. You are the blossoming flower that grew from seeds planted with intention and love, nurtured through life's seasons of change.

Holistic self-care is your journey, your rhythm, and your sanctuary. It's a path of embracing who you are, flaws and all, and nurturing your whole self—body, mind, and spirit. It's not about perfection but about progress and presence. You are already enough, already worthy, and already beautiful. Let this chapter serve as a reminder that taking care of yourself is not selfish—it's essential. It's how you bloom.

So, take a moment to honor the path you've walked, the lessons you've learned, and the incredible person you are becoming. Continue to plant those seeds, tend to your garden, and let your beauty and strength flourish. You deserve every moment of joy, peace, and fulfillment that comes from caring for yourself. This is your celebration—your reminder that the most important relationship in your life is the one you have with yourself. You are worthy of the time, the effort, and the love. Always.

CHAPTER 6
IMAGERY
THE POWER OF HEALING THROUGH THE MIND'S EYE

When it comes to true healing, the body and mind are deeply intertwined. While we often think of medicine and therapy as the keys to physical health, the power of our imagination is an untapped resource that can shape the way we experience and respond to pain, stress, and even medical treatments. **Imagery**, the practice of visualizing calming and positive scenes or sensations, taps into this natural mind-body connection, creating real changes in our physiology and emotions.

Let me share a story from my own work in a clinical setting. There was a patient, visibly tense, about to receive an IV. She'd been through this process before and had developed a real fear of the needle. I could see her shoulders tightening, her hands clenching the armrest, and her breathing becoming shallow. That's when I suggested something simple yet profound. I asked her to close her eyes and imagine herself in her favorite place—a quiet beach, the sun warming her skin, waves gently lapping at her feet. I described each detail, encouraging her to breathe deeply and feel the comfort of that imagined space. By the time we were ready for the IV, her grip had softened, and her breathing was steady. When the needle went in, she barely flinched.

This wasn't magic—it was the power of imagery in action. When we consciously use our imagination, we invite the mind to influence our body's response to stress, pain, and anxiety. Imagery can make such a difference that it's now widely recognized as a complementary tool in clinical settings. But how, exactly, does it work?

HOW IMAGERY WORKS: THE SCIENCE BEHIND THE MIND-BODY CONNECTION

The mind doesn't always distinguish between what is real and what is imagined. When we visualize a relaxing scene or a positive outcome, our brain responds as if it's really happening. This response triggers a cascade of physiological changes through the nervous system, impacting our heart rate, blood pressure, and even our immune response.

Here's why imagery has such powerful effects:

- **Blood Flow and Muscle Relaxation:** When we're anxious or in pain, the body goes into a "fight-or-flight" mode, which tightens muscles and constricts blood vessels. Imagery, by helping us envision a calming experience, activates the body's parasympathetic nervous system—essentially our "rest and digest" system. This activation dilates blood vessels, improving blood flow and allowing tense muscles to relax. It's like giving your body permission to let go.

- **Heart Rate and Blood Pressure Regulation:** During stressful or painful moments, our heart races and blood pressure spikes as part of the body's natural stress response. But when we engage in imagery, the body interprets these positive scenes as a signal that it's safe to calm down. This, in turn, slows the heart rate and lowers blood pressure, creating a sense of calm. The body is reassured, "You're safe here. You don't need to be on high alert."

- **Enhanced Immune Function:** Believe it or not, positive mental imagery can boost immune function. Studies have shown that visualizing scenes of gratitude or appreciation creates what's known as "physiologic coherence," a state where the body's systems synchronize and work more efficiently. This state of harmony is associated with a stronger immune response, likely because stress hormones that weaken immunity are reduced.
- **Pain Management:** Imagery can reshape our perception of pain by helping the mind interpret it differently. When we visualize pain as something that can be changed—by giving it a color, a shape, or even shrinking it in our mind—the brain perceives the pain as less intense. This phenomenon occurs because imagery helps shift the brain's focus away from pain signals, reducing their intensity.

GUIDED IMAGERY IN PRACTICE: STORIES FROM THE CLINICAL SETTING

In clinical settings, I've witnessed the impact of imagery on patients preparing for procedures. One elderly man had to undergo a knee replacement surgical procedure, and he was visibly anxious. His hands shook, and he expressed his fear to me, worried about the pain and the recovery. I took a few minutes to guide him through a simple imagery exercise. I asked him to imagine his favorite place—a serene cabin in the woods where he could smell the pine trees and hear the gentle rustle of leaves. As he breathed deeply and visualized, his muscles visibly relaxed, and his face softened. By the time the doctor was ready, he was far more at ease, and he later told me that his recovery felt smoother than he had expected.

Imagery isn't just a passive daydream. It's a powerful, scientifically-backed method of engaging the mind in a way that influences the body's physical state. Imagine preparing for a routine shot and feeling your anxiety build up. Instead of focusing on the needle, you take a few deep breaths, close your eyes, and visualize a calming place—a peaceful forest, the warmth of the sun, a soft breeze on your face. By the time the needle goes in, you're so focused on your imagined scene that the experience feels entirely different. This isn't magic; it's the brain's ability to redirect focus and reduce physical tension.

THE HEALING BENEFITS OF IMAGERY

The benefits of imagery extend far beyond the doctor's office. Imagery can be incorporated into our daily lives to help manage stress, pain, and emotional strain. Let's explore some common uses:

1. **Daily Stress Relief:** Many people use imagery in the morning or before bed to prepare for or unwind from the day. Visualizing a calm, safe place helps activate the parasympathetic nervous system, reducing stress and promoting relaxation.
2. **Managing Fear and Worry:** For those dealing with ongoing anxiety or worry, dedicating 10–20 minutes to "Worry and Fear Imagery" each day can make a huge difference. Picture each worry as a feather or a leaf, gently floating away on a breeze. This simple exercise can help release the grip of anxiety, reminding the mind that worries are not permanent.
3. **Pain Management:** In pain management, imagery is used to visualize pain as something that can be changed—giving it a shape or color, imagining it shrinking or softening. This helps patients perceive pain as less overwhelming, a technique that has shown effectiveness in people with chronic conditions.

CLINICAL EFFECTIVENESS: THE RESEARCH-BACKED POWER OF IMAGERY

The impact of imagery is so profound that it has been studied in various clinical settings. Research shows that imagery can increase blood flow, enhance immune responses, control heart rate, and aid in wound healing. Imagery isn't just "in your head"—it creates measurable physical effects.

For example, studies using MRI have shown that when people imagine a physical sensation, such as tasting a lemon, their brain responds as if they are actually experiencing it. The same principle applies to healing and relaxation. When we imagine positive sensations, the brain releases endorphins and other feel-good chemicals, creating a genuine, physical sense of relief and calm.

IMAGERY TECHNIQUES YOU CAN TRY

Here are a few techniques you can incorporate into your daily routine:

1. **Basic Relaxation Imagery:** Close your eyes, take a few deep breaths, and imagine yourself in a place that feels safe and comfortable. Let yourself become absorbed in the sounds, sights, and sensations around you. Use this technique when feeling anxious or overwhelmed.
2. **Worry and Fear Imagery:** Visualize each worry as something small and manageable—a pebble, a leaf, or even a cloud. Let it drift away, reminding yourself that you don't have to hold onto it. Repeat this daily for a grounding effect.
3. **Pain Management Imagery:** Focus on the area of discomfort and imagine it as an object with color, shape, and size. Then, mentally shrink or soften it, noticing any changes in sensation. This can be useful for chronic pain or moments of acute discomfort.

CONCLUSION: IMAGERY AS A PATHWAY TO HOLISTIC HEALTH

Imagery is a powerful tool that brings the mind and body into harmony. It's a way to tap into the body's natural healing mechanisms through the mind's focus and intention. By practicing imagery, you can cultivate a sense of inner strength, resilience, and peace. It's not only a method for coping with pain or stress; it's a lifelong skill for nurturing wellness.

Imagery reminds us that, even in the midst of pain or anxiety, we have the power to change our experience. By connecting with our inner landscape, we engage in a form of healing that reaches beyond medicine, fostering a balance of mind, body, and spirit.

CHAPTER 7

THE ART OF RELAXATION

BREATHING YOUR WAY TO HEALTH,
WELLNESS, AND BEAUTY

Relaxation—such a simple concept, yet for many of us, truly letting go of stress can feel as unattainable as a distant dream. We are constantly rushing from one thing to another, juggling responsibilities at work, managing things at home, and trying to squeeze in self-care whenever we can. But imagine if we could turn relaxation into a tool we carry with us, accessible anytime, anywhere. That is what this chapter is all about: empowering you with practical relaxation techniques that are easy to integrate into your life and can make a meaningful difference in your health, wellness, and beauty. When we talk about beauty, we often overlook that stress is one of its biggest enemies. Stress shows up in unexpected places—our skin, our hair, even our posture. It can trigger inflammation, accelerate aging, and drain the glow from our faces. Incorporating relaxation into your daily routine is not just good for the soul; it's like giving yourself an internal spa day, a reset that reflects on the outside too. Let us dive into some powerful, portable techniques to help.

THE POWER OF BREATH: TECHNIQUES YOU CAN TAKE ANYWHERE

When it comes to relaxation, breathing is our unsung hero. Not only does it work wonders in calming the mind, but it also has a profound effect on our entire system—lowering blood pressure, reducing stress hormones, and even enhancing our immune function. And the best part? You do not need a yoga mat, special gear, or time blocked out in your calendar. Just your breath.

1. Mindful Breathing Script for Everyday Moments

This is one of my favorite go-to breathing techniques, perfect for those small pockets of time we usually waste scrolling through our phones. I often used this with patients who were feeling anxious before a procedure, and it was incredible to see the shift it created in them.

Script:
Breathing in, I am aware of my breath entering.
Breathing out, I am letting go of any tension.
In: I am calm.
Out: I am at peace.

Try this for a few minutes, whether you are waiting in line, before a meeting, or even during your morning coffee. Breathing does not just supply oxygen to your cells; it's like a mini massage for your nervous system, helping you carry a sense of calm wherever you go.

2. Walking Meditation with Breath

Walking meditation is another technique I have found incredibly grounding—for myself and my patients alike. When I was helping a patient prepare for an IV, for instance, guiding them to focus on their breath with each step gave them something to focus on other than their fear. It is also a beautiful practice for those days when you're struggling to sit still. Here's how to do it:

Begin by standing tall. As you step forward with your left foot, breathe in slowly.
Take another step, breathing out.
Repeat, synchronizing your steps with your breaths.

It does not matter where you're walking—in a garden, down the hospital corridor, or even around your kitchen. Each step is a moment of peace you are gifting yourself. This practice has helped me personally on stressful days and is something I return to when I need to find balance. Every step is a reminder to slow down, breathe, and be fully present.

3. Guided Visualization for Deep Relaxation

Imagine you are guiding your breath to parts of your body that feel tense or tired. When I first used this technique on a patient who was nervous before surgery, the results were almost magical. I had them visualize their breath traveling to tense spots: their shoulders, neck, even the muscles around their eyes—releasing tension with each exhale. This can be done anytime you feel the weight of the world building up. **Here's a simple visualization script:

1. Close your eyes.
2. Breathe in; imagine the air moving through your chest and reaching those tense spots.
3. Exhale, feeling the tension release and drift away.
4. Continue this for a few breaths, mentally telling each area to soften and relax. This technique not only calms your mind but can also physically relieve tension, helping you look and feel more refreshed.

Here's how you can incorporate the scientific reasoning for each practice into the relaxation techniques section while keeping it clear, engaging, and relevant for your audience:

PRACTICAL TIPS FOR INTEGRATING RELAXATION INTO YOUR LIFE

Let's talk about making relaxation part of your everyday life. No elaborate rituals or spa days are needed (though we'll take those when we can get them!). These techniques are your on-the-go wellness kit, supported by science to ensure they're not only practical but also effective.

1. While Cooking or Cleaning

- **What to Do:** As you chop vegetables, stir a pot, or fold laundry, take slow, deliberate breaths. Inhale deeply through your nose, hold for a moment, and exhale fully through your mouth.
- **Why It Works:** Deep breathing reduces cortisol, the body's primary stress hormone, by activating the parasympathetic nervous system (your "rest and digest" mode). This helps lower your heart rate and blood pressure, making these everyday chores surprisingly calming.

2. Morning Wake-Up Breathing

- **What to Do:** Before stepping out of bed, place one hand on your belly and the other on your chest. Take five slow, deep breaths, letting your stomach rise on the inhale and fall on the exhale.
- **Why It Works:** Morning breathing engages the diaphragm, stimulating the vagus nerve. This kickstarts your parasympathetic response, helping you start the day with calm energy and a clear mind. It's like a gentle reset button for your nervous system.

3. Daily Breath Breaks

- **What to Do:** Set a timer on your phone for a one-minute breathing session three times a day. Close your eyes, breathe in deeply for a count of four, hold for four, and exhale for six.

- **Why It Works:** Known as "4-4-6 breathing," this technique lowers cortisol and increases oxygen flow to the brain. It not only reduces stress but also enhances focus and energy, making it a quick pick-me-up during a hectic day.

4. Sitting in Your Car

- **What to Do:** Before stepping out for a big meeting, job interview, or stressful errand, sit in your car and try box breathing. Inhale for four counts, hold for four, exhale for four, and hold for four. Repeat four times.
- **Why It Works:** Box breathing stabilizes your autonomic nervous system, balancing stress hormones and reducing feelings of anxiety. It's often used by Navy SEALs to stay calm in high-pressure situations— a testament to its effectiveness.

5. Before an Important Interview

- **What to Do:** Practice progressive muscle relaxation (PMR). Starting at your toes, tense each muscle group for five seconds, then release. Work your way up to your neck and shoulders.
- **Why It Works:** PMR helps reduce overall muscle tension while increasing awareness of stress-prone areas. The release phase signals your body to shift into a relaxed state, leaving you feeling grounded and ready to face challenges.

6. Guided Visualization

- **What to Do:** Close your eyes and picture a place where you feel safe and happy, like a serene beach or a cozy cabin. Imagine the sights, sounds, and sensations

vividly. Spend 2–5 minutes fully immersed in this scene.
- **Why It Works:** Visualization reduces activity in the amygdala, the brain's fear center, while boosting endorphin production. It helps calm anxiety, improve mood, and even lower physical tension.

7. Evening Wind-Down Routine

- **What to Do:** Dedicate five minutes before bed to mindful breathing. Sit in a quiet space, light a candle if you'd like, and focus on slow inhales and exhales. Pair this with gratitude by reflecting on one positive moment from your day.
- **Why It Works:**Slow breathing reduces cortisol and increases melatonin, the hormone responsible for regulating sleep. Gratitude has been shown to boost serotonin levels, promoting a sense of peace and well-being.

By understanding the science behind these practices, you'll not only find them easier to incorporate into your life but also appreciate their profound impact on your mind and body. These small yet powerful techniques are your tools for cultivating calm and beauty from within—accessible anytime, anywhere.

MEDITATION FOR RELAXATION AND HEALING

Meditation might sound like something only monks in serene mountaintop monasteries do, but trust me—it's far more accessible than that. Think of it as "me-time" for your brain. It's not about emptying your mind or sitting cross-legged for hours; it's about giving yourself a moment to breathe and let go. And the benefits? Oh, they're amazing—lower blood pressure, a stronger immune system, and even a higher pain tolerance. (Translation: it's like a secret superpower!)

THE RELAXATION RESPONSE MEDITATION

This simple, stress-busting technique by Dr. Herbert Benson is a game-changer. You pick a calming word or phrase—something like "peace" or "calm"—and silently repeat it in your mind. When distractions pop up (because they will), just gently guide your focus back. It's not about getting it perfect—it's about showing up for yourself.

Here's the best part: just a few minutes a day can make a huge difference. Whether you're in a chaotic household or sneaking in a quick break at work, this little practice can bring you back to center.

WALKING MEDITATION: TAKING EACH STEP WITH PEACE

For those of us who can't sit still for long (no shame—we're movers!), walking meditation is a fantastic option. Picture this: you're walking, but instead of mentally running through your to-do list, you focus on your steps and your breath. It's like turning a simple stroll into a mini spa session for your mind.

Here's how it works: inhale over three steps, exhale over the next three. Feel the ground beneath your feet and notice your breath moving through you. Bonus points if you can squeeze this in while walking to grab your morning coffee or heading back to your car after work.

COMPASSION MEDITATION: CULTIVATING KINDNESS FROM WITHIN

This one's a heartwarmer, inspired by Christian teachings about love and compassion. Start by sitting quietly and tuning into God's presence. Then, repeat phrases like, "May I feel God's peace. May I be filled with His love. May I extend His grace to others." It's like a spiritual hug for your soul.

Once you've centered yourself, extend these loving thoughts to others—your family, friends, and yes, even that person who cut you off in traffic. (They need grace too, right?) This practice not only relaxes your heart but also fills you with a sense of connection and forgiveness, easing emotional stress along the way.

RESTORATIVE YOGA: SURRENDERING INTO PEACE

If you've ever thought, "I just need to hit pause on life for a moment," restorative yoga is your best friend. This isn't your typical yoga class where you're twisting yourself into a pretzel—it's all about comfort and stillness. With props like blankets and bolsters, you settle into fully supported poses and just… let go.

Imagine lying in a cozy nest of blankets, breathing deeply, and feeling all the tension melt away. It's like a nap, but better because you're consciously unwinding. It's the perfect antidote to a hectic day.

CREATING A PERSONAL HEALING SPACE: YOUR SANCTUARY OF CALM

You don't need a fancy spa or a Pinterest-worthy setup to relax (though if you have one, go for it!). All you need is a small corner in your home that feels like you. Add a candle, a soft blanket, maybe a plant or two—voilà, your personal oasis.

This little sanctuary becomes your go-to spot for unwinding after a long day. Whether you're reading, sipping tea, or just sitting in stillness, having a dedicated space can make relaxation feel like a daily luxury instead of an occasional treat.

By weaving these practices into your day, you're not just managing stress—you're treating yourself to moments of peace that ripple through every part of your life. Relaxation isn't a luxury; it's a gift you give yourself. So, take a deep breath, try one of these techniques, and remember: even a few minutes of calm can brighten your whole day.

And hey, if all else fails, there's always chocolate and a cozy blanket waiting in your healing space!

THE BEAUTY OF RELAXATION – HOW IT MAKES YOU GLOW

Relaxation isn't just for calming your mind; it's your secret beauty treatment. When you're relaxed, your skin glows, your posture improves, and your natural vibrancy shines through. By reducing stress hormones like cortisol—which can cause dull skin and breakouts—you create the perfect conditions for your beauty to flourish. And the best part? Relaxation is free, available anytime, and its only side effect is undeniable radiance.

When you prioritize relaxation, you're nourishing yourself from the inside out. Each moment of calm you create is like a gift to your health, wellness, and beauty.

WRAPPING IT UP: MAKING RELAXATION A LIFESTYLE

Relaxation doesn't have to mean a full day at the spa (although that's always welcome!). It's about weaving moments of calm and presence into your everyday life. Whether it's a few deep breaths while sitting in your car, a quiet meditation before bed, or showing yourself compassion during a tough moment, these small acts add up.

Relaxation is essential—it's the secret ingredient that keeps you grounded, resilient, and yes, radiant. When we embrace relaxation as a daily practice, we're better equipped to navigate life's challenges with grace and confidence.

So, take a moment for yourself. Breathe deeply, smile, and let the beauty of relaxation become part of your lifestyle. You deserve this time to recharge, reconnect, and shine—inside and out.

CHAPTER 8
BODY AND MIND IN HARMONY
THE FOUNDATION OF TRUE WELLNESS

The connection between the body and mind is more than just a wellness buzzword—it's the foundation of true health and vitality. Our thoughts, emotions, and physical state are deeply intertwined, creating a powerful feedback loop that shapes our overall well-being. Whether it's the tension in your shoulders from a stressful day or the boost of energy you feel after an inspiring moment, your body and mind are constantly communicating. Understanding and nurturing this connection allows you to not only feel your best but also radiate confidence and balance in every aspect of your life.

A CONVERSATION BETWEEN BODY AND MIND

Picture this: Your body and mind are like two best friends. Some days, they're perfectly in sync, finishing each other's sentences. Other days, it's like they're speaking completely different languages. But one thing's for sure—they're always talking to each other.

Let's talk stress—a prime example of this dialogue. Imagine you've planned a perfectly productive day: a morning workout, a spotless house, deadlines crushed at work, and maybe even some "me time" before bed. Then, real life happens.

You get a call from school that your child isn't feeling well and needs to be picked up immediately. Now, you're juggling comforting a sick kid, rescheduling meetings, and trying to squeeze in your never-ending to-do list. Before you know it, stress takes over. Cortisol, the infamous stress hormone, kicks in, and your body reacts like it's under attack.

Your heart races, your shoulders tighten, and your stomach starts doing its own performance—think upset, bloating, or that gnawing, uneasy feeling. To make matters worse, your skin chimes in with a breakout, as if adding its own commentary to the chaos.

Now flip the script. Imagine an afternoon where everything falls into place. You're sipping tea while the sunlight streams through the window, or you're at a yoga class, soaking in the calm energy around you. In these moments, your body says, "Ah, finally!" Blood pressure eases, your breathing slows, and your skin? It's practically glowing with gratitude.

This constant back-and-forth between your body and mind is more than fascinating—it's empowering. It's a reminder that even amidst chaos, we have the tools to pause, listen, and respond.

So, the next time your stomach feels uneasy or your jaw feels tight, pause. Ask yourself: What's my body trying to tell me? It might just be asking for a moment to breathe, a break to reset, or a little love and care to restore balance.

THE POWER TRIO: NERVOUS, ENDOCRINE, AND IMMUNE SYSTEMS

Imagine your nervous system as the body's command center, running everything from typing a text to processing your late-night thoughts. Then there's the endocrine system, your body's hormone headquarters, managing mood, metabolism, and how you handle stress. Finally, we have the immune system, your ever-vigilant bodyguard, warding off illnesses and keeping you strong. Together, these three systems form an intricate network, constantly chatting and collaborating to determine how you feel—both physically and emotionally.

But what happens when life gets overwhelming? Picture this: Your nervous system, always on the lookout for potential threats, shoots a quick message to the endocrine system, saying, "Sound the alarm!" In response, your endocrine system releases stress hormones like cortisol and adrenaline, preparing your body to either fight the threat or flee from it. This "fight or flight" mode is incredibly useful when you're dodging real danger—say, a bear in the woods. But let's be honest, most of us aren't running from bears. Instead, we're racing against deadlines, handling sick kids, or juggling endless to-do lists.

When stress becomes chronic, it's like the emergency alarm in your body gets stuck in the "on" position. Constantly pumping out stress hormones takes a toll—disrupting your sleep, weakening your immune defenses, and leaving you feeling drained. Chronic stress isn't just in your head; it impacts your body in profound ways.

NEUROPEPTIDES: THE BODY'S EMOTIONAL MESSENGERS

Now, let's dive into the fascinating world of **neuropeptides**—those tiny molecules that act as emotional messengers, connecting your brain and body. These little powerhouses are produced by neurons in the brain and cells throughout your body, delivering messages about how you feel. Think of them as the texts flying back and forth in a group chat between your brain, your gut, and your muscles.

When you're happy, neuropeptides send signals of joy and calm, helping you relax and feel at ease. But when stress creeps in, these same messengers transmit distress signals that tighten your muscles or churn your stomach into knots. Ever felt a "gut feeling" about something? That's neuropeptides at work, translating your emotional experiences into physical sensations.

Here's where it gets even more fascinating: most of the receptors for neuropeptides are in your gut. No wonder the digestive system is often called your "second brain." It's why anxiety can make your stomach act up or why excitement can send butterflies fluttering through your belly.

By understanding the role of neuropeptides, you can start to see how your emotions influence your physical state—and why managing stress is so essential for overall wellness. It's all connected, from the knot in your stomach during a tough day to the calm you feel after a walk in nature or a heartfelt laugh.

HOW NEUROPEPTIDES KEEP US FEELING GOOD (OR NOT!)

Imagine you're preparing for a big meeting or presentation. You might feel nervous, right? Well, your brain releases neuropeptides related to stress, which then activate your adrenal glands to release cortisol. This creates physical symptoms like sweaty palms, a racing heart, or that anxious feeling in the pit of your stomach. But here's the amazing part: neuropeptides don't only handle stress; they're also behind those positive emotions we crave.

Take **endorphins**, for example. These "feel-good" neuropeptides are released when we exercise, laugh, or even eat chocolate (yes, it's science!). They help relieve pain, boost mood, and give us that little "runner's high" after a good workout. And let's not forget **oxytocin**—the "love hormone" released during bonding activities like hugging, spending time with loved ones, or even petting your dog. It's the chemical that makes us feel warm, connected, and safe.

In other words, neuropeptides are our body's way of translating emotions into physical sensations. When we feel happy, connected, or calm, neuropeptides like oxytocin and endorphins help reinforce those feelings, creating a "good vibes" feedback loop. And when we're stressed, it's the opposite; stress-related neuropeptides keep us in that tense, on-edge state.

So, how can we make the most of this body-mind connection in our daily lives?

START WITH YOUR THOUGHTS – THEY'RE MORE POWERFUL THAN YOU THINK

Our thoughts are incredibly potent. As a nurse, I've seen how deeply stress and negativity can impact patients' health—not just mentally but physically. When we're under stress, the body reacts in ways that go far beyond the surface: inflammation increases, the immune system weakens, and hormones spiral out of balance. This isn't just a mental exercise; it's happening at a cellular level.

I remember one patient, a young woman, who came to our clinic for help managing her chronic migraines. Traditional treatments weren't working, and her stress levels were off the charts. We introduced her to biofeedback as a way to bring awareness to her body's responses. By learning how her heart rate and muscle tension spiked with stress, she could begin to take control. Using guided breathing techniques and positive affirmations, she started noticing small but meaningful changes —not just in her migraines but in her overall well-being.

Positive affirmations, gratitude journaling, and reframing negative thoughts aren't just "feel-good" suggestions—they're proven tools for holistic health. Research shows that maintaining a positive outlook can reduce inflammation, lower blood pressure, and even strengthen the immune system. It's like giving your cells a little daily pep talk.

Pro Tip: Next time you're overwhelmed, pause for a deep breath and say something kind to yourself. A simple "I'm doing my best, and that's enough" can work wonders. You'd be amazed at how quickly your body follows your mind's lead.

NEUROPLASTICITY – YES, YOU CAN TEACH YOUR BRAIN NEW TRICKS!

For years, we believed the brain was fixed, unable to change after childhood. Thankfully, science proved that wrong. Neuroplasticity—the brain's ability to rewire itself—shows that we can teach our brains new ways of thinking and reacting, no matter our age.

I once worked with a middle-aged patient recovering from heart surgery. She had a habit of responding to stress with unhealthy comfort foods, which only exacerbated her health issues. Together, we used biofeedback to help her identify the early physical signs of stress—like a tightening chest or shallow breathing. Then, we introduced small, manageable alternatives: pausing for deep breaths, drinking a glass of water, or going for a short walk instead of reaching for chips. Over time, those small shifts became her new normal. Watching her regain control of her habits—and her health—was incredible.

The best part? This kind of transformation isn't limited to biofeedback sessions. Whether through mindfulness, meditation, or even simple daily practices, you can create new pathways in your brain that promote calmness and resilience. It's all about consistency.

Try This: The next time you feel the urge to react to stress in an unhealthy way, pause. Take three deep breaths, in through your nose and out through your mouth. It's a small act, but it's the first step in teaching your brain a new trick.

EMOTIONAL RESPONSES – LISTENING TO YOUR BODY'S SIGNALS

Our emotions don't just live in our minds—they manifest throughout our bodies. As a nurse, I've seen how emotions can become physical signals: tense shoulders during anxiety, a heavy chest during grief, or butterflies in the stomach from excitement. These aren't random—they're your body's way of processing feelings.

One patient of mine, newly diagnosed with a chronic illness, would often come to appointments with severe shoulder pain. She was convinced it was unrelated to her stress, but her body was telling a different story. Through biofeedback and mindful awareness practices, she learned to identify the connection between her emotions and physical sensations. By addressing her anxiety with deep breathing and progressive muscle relaxation, the tension in her shoulders began to ease.

Emotions are not inconveniences; they're messages. Ignoring them only makes the signals louder, often manifesting as physical pain or discomfort. Listening to those signals and responding with care—whether it's stretching, meditating, or simply naming the emotion—can make a world of difference.

Pro Tip: The next time you feel tightness or discomfort, ask yourself: What emotion am I holding here? Sometimes, just acknowledging it can start the healing process.

BRINGING IT ALL TOGETHER: YOUR MIND AS YOUR ALLY

By understanding the power of our thoughts, leveraging neuroplasticity, and tuning into our body's emotional signals, we can take charge of our well-being. Whether it's through biofeedback, mindfulness, or just small daily habits, we have the tools to reshape how we respond to life's challenges.

Remember, your mind isn't working against you—it's your greatest ally. When you treat it with kindness and intention, it will reward you with strength, resilience, and peace. And isn't that a relationship worth investing in?

PRACTICAL TIPS FOR TAPPING INTO THE BODY-MIND CONNECTION

You might notice that some of these techniques, like mindful breathing and walking meditation, will be described in more detail in later chapters. For now, I want to highlight them in the context of the powerful connection between body and mind. These practices are foundational, and understanding their role here will help you see how they influence other aspects of wellness and beauty as we explore further. Let's dive into how these simple techniques strengthen the intricate relationship between your body and mind. They are small but powerful steps toward feeling your best.

Mindful Breathing: The One-Minute Reset

Life can feel like a whirlwind sometimes, with our minds spinning in a million directions. That's where mindful breathing steps in—a simple yet powerful tool to ground yourself. It's easy: inhale deeply, hold for a moment, and then exhale slowly. Repeat a few times, and just like that, you feel calmer and more centered.

Why does it matter? Mindful breathing is like a mini vacation for your body. It helps reset your nervous system, lowers cortisol levels (that infamous stress hormone), and provides a much-needed moment of calm amidst the chaos. Think of it as hitting the pause button—a quick yet effective way to remind your body and mind that it's okay to slow down.

Meditation for Healing: A Simple Reset for Your Mind and Body

Meditation might sound intimidating, but it's really just about creating a little space for yourself to breathe and reset. Forget the image of hours of silence or complicated poses—you can benefit from just a few minutes a day.

Why meditate? It's like a mental reset button. It helps reduce stress, improves focus, and even lowers blood pressure. Plus, it's the perfect antidote for those "mom moments" when life feels overwhelming. Just five minutes while waiting for coffee or before bed can be transformative.

Walking Meditation: A Calming Practice in Motion

If sitting still feels impossible (we've all been there!), walking meditation is a great alternative. It combines movement and mindfulness, making it a practical choice for busy days.

How It Works:

1. **Start With Intent:** Pick a quiet place like your backyard, a park, or even your living room.
2. **Sync Your Steps and Breath:** Walk slowly, inhaling as one foot steps forward and exhaling with the next.
3. **Engage Your Senses:** Notice the feeling of your shoes on the ground, the rhythm of your breath, and the sounds around you.

Walking meditation is perfect for multitaskers—it lets you meditate and move simultaneously, grounding yourself while still getting things done. Bonus points if you can step outside for fresh air—it's an instant mood booster.

Actionable Tips to Weave Meditation Into Daily Life

1. Start Small and Stay Consistent

Begin with just 2-5 minutes a day and build from there. Even short sessions can have long-lasting benefits.

2. Use Guided Meditations

Apps like Calm, Headspace, or Insight Timer are great tools for beginners, offering quick, tailored meditations for stress relief, sleep, or confidence-building.

3. Pair Meditation With Daily Activities

Meditate while waiting for coffee, during your skincare routine, or even at red lights during your commute.

4. Incorporate Visualization

Imagine yourself in a serene place—walking through a lush forest, sitting by the ocean, or floating on a calm lake. Visualization enhances relaxation and engages your creative mind.

5. Focus on Gratitude

During meditation, reflect on one or two things you're grateful for. It's a simple way to shift your mindset and bring positivity into your practice.

These techniques aren't just about calming the mind—they're about creating a stronger connection between your body and mind. They're small, practical steps that anyone can take to create a ripple effect of wellness throughout their day. Remember, it's not about perfection; it's about progress. Whether it's a few mindful breaths or a quick walking meditation, each moment you take for yourself is a step toward greater balance and well-being.

Why Women Should Prioritize Meditation

Between juggling careers, family, and personal goals, women often put their own well-being last. Meditation is a simple yet powerful tool to reclaim moments of peace and clarity amidst the chaos. It doesn't require perfection—just a commitment to showing up for yourself daily. Whether you're sitting in stillness, walking through nature, or repeating affirmations during your shower, meditation helps anchor you, reminding you that amidst life's noise, your inner calm is always within reach.

CREATE YOUR PERSONAL SANCTUARY: A SPACE JUST FOR YOU

Your surroundings have a huge impact on how you feel, so why not carve out a little slice of peace in your home? It doesn't have to be extravagant—a cozy chair by the window, a nook filled with your favorite books, or even a quiet corner of your bedroom can do the trick. Add a few calming elements like a soft blanket, a scented candle, or a plant. This can be your refuge when life feels overwhelming.

Why have a sanctuary? Because having a space that's yours —a spot that reminds you to pause and breathe—can work wonders for your mental and emotional health. Over time, your brain will associate this spot with relaxation and comfort, making it easier to slip into a calmer state whenever you're there. It's like your personal retreat, no travel required.

Pro Tip for Moms: Share your sanctuary rules with your family—maybe it's "Mom's 15-minute time-out zone." Trust me, they'll respect it when they see how much calmer and happier you are after taking that time for yourself.

COMPASSIONATE SELF-TALK: BE YOUR OWN BEST FRIEND

Let's get real—most of us are way too hard on ourselves. Would you ever tell a friend, "Wow, you really messed that up"? Of course not! So why do we let that inner critic run wild? It's time to flip the script. When you catch yourself being overly harsh, pause and ask: What would I say to a friend in this situation? Now, say that to yourself instead.

Why self-kindness matters: Because when we treat ourselves with compassion, our body gets the memo that it's okay to relax. Studies show that self-compassion can actually lower stress and improve overall well-being. It's like pressing a reset button for your soul, helping you recharge and find balance from within.

A Quick Exercise: Next time you're feeling overwhelmed, place a hand on your heart and say something kind to yourself. It might feel awkward at first, but with practice, it becomes a powerful tool for calming your mind and boosting your confidence.

Example: After an argument with a friend or family member, when self-doubt creeps in, place your hand on your heart and say, "I am human, and it's okay to make mistakes. I choose to learn and grow from this."

Lighthearted Reminder: If you catch yourself spiraling into self-criticism, imagine your inner critic wearing a silly outfit—like a clown hat or mismatched socks. It's hard to take harsh thoughts seriously when you're picturing that!

Example: You're stressing over forgetting something important. Picture your inner critic wearing mismatched shoes—one cowboy boot and one flip-flop—and trying to look serious. You might even chuckle.

By creating a sanctuary and practicing self-compassion, you're not just taking care of your mental health—you're giving yourself permission to thrive. These small, intentional acts send a message: I am worthy of peace, kindness, and joy.

MOVE YOUR BODY: BEYOND THE GYM— FINDING JOY IN MOVEMENT

We all know exercise is good for us, but let's think beyond just building muscles or ticking off gym sessions. Movement is about so much more—it's a way to nurture your mind and body, release tension, and flood your system with those magical "feel-good" chemicals, endorphins. Think of it as a natural, free boost of happiness!

Why Move?

Because moving your body keeps those neuropeptides flowing —helping you stay mentally sharp, emotionally balanced, and physically energized. It's not about how intense the workout is; it's about finding ways to move that bring you joy and leave you feeling uplifted.

- **A Walk Around the Block:** Perfect for clearing your mind after a stressful day. Bonus points if you can soak up a little sunshine.
- **Yoga:** A calming practice that combines stretching and mindfulness, perfect for unwinding after a long day or kickstarting your morning with clarity.
- **Dance It Out:** Put on your favorite playlist and have a living room dance party. No one's watching—so go wild!
- **Stretching Breaks:** Even a few minutes of stretching during work or household chores can ease tension and reset your focus.
- **Chasing Kids Around the Yard:** Who says playtime isn't a workout? It's a fun, heart-pumping way to bond and stay active.

Finding Joy in Movement

The key is to reframe how you think about exercise. It's not a chore or another box to check—it's a gift to yourself. Discover what kind of movement feels good for you and fits your lifestyle. Some days it might be a brisk walk; other days, it's a few deep stretches before bed.

So, lace up those sneakers, roll out that yoga mat, or press play on your favorite song. Whatever movement looks like for you, make it yours—because when you move your body, you're not just exercising; you're energizing your life!

CONNECTION AND LAUGHTER: A FAMILY AFFAIR

There's nothing quite like a good laugh to lift your spirits. Whether it's gathering around the dinner table to share funny stories, playing a silly game with your kids, or hearing their wildly imaginative jokes, these moments are more than just fun —they're medicine for the soul. Laughter helps release **oxytocin**, the "bonding hormone," which not only strengthens our immunity but also naturally melts away stress.

Why connect and laugh? Because we're wired for connection, and laughter is one of the simplest ways to build it. It reminds us that joy is contagious and that even in the busiest seasons of life, small, lighthearted moments matter. Picture this: you're playing a board game with your family, and someone makes an outrageous move that has everyone laughing until their sides hurt. That's not just entertainment—it's creating memories and nurturing your well-being.

When you take the time to meet up with friends or loved ones, let yourself laugh, relax, and be present. It's not just good for your mood—it's good for your health. And don't overlook the power of these small but meaningful connections in bringing balance and joy to your everyday life.

By incorporating small, mindful practices like connection and laughter into your routine, you're not just managing stress—you're nurturing your whole self. When your body and mind work in harmony, you'll see the benefits not just in how you feel but also in how you carry yourself and connect with the world around you.

Remember, change doesn't have to be drastic to make a difference. Start small. Maybe it's a weekly game night, a daily moment of gratitude, or simply choosing to smile when things feel heavy. Wellness is found in these little moments, as much as in the grand ones.

So take a deep breath, enjoy the silly moments, and let yourself savor each step of this journey. You're not striving for perfection—you're creating a life that feels balanced, joyful, and beautifully you. You've got this!

A PERSONAL NOTE

As a nurse, I've witnessed firsthand the profound impact of the **body-mind connection**. I recall working with a patient who was nearly paralyzed with anxiety before a procedure. Her hands trembled, and her heartbeat was racing. Together, we practiced deep breathing—a simple in-and-out rhythm—and I encouraged her to silently repeat a calming phrase like, I am safe, and I can do this.

By the time we began, her hands had steadied, her heartbeat had slowed, and her entire demeanor had softened. It was remarkable to see how a small, intentional pause could transform her experience—not just mentally but physically too.

Moments like these serve as powerful reminders: we all have the ability to influence our own well-being. The **body-mind connection** isn't just a lofty concept—it's a tangible, practical tool you can use daily. And the best part? You don't need a medical degree or special training to benefit. All it takes is a willingness to pause, breathe deeply, and tune into your body's natural wisdom.

In a world that often pulls us in a million directions, remember this: the path to beauty and wellness starts with listening to yourself. You have everything you need within you—just give yourself the time and space to connect.

MAKING THE BODY-MIND CONNECTION PART OF YOUR LIFE

Incorporating the body-mind connection into your daily life doesn't require hours of practice. It's about small, intentional acts that, over time, lead to lasting change. Start your day with a few deep breaths, take mindful breaks, or end the night with a short meditation. Every little moment helps.

The body-mind connection is a gift—a bridge between your inner thoughts and outer health. By honoring this connection, you're nurturing not only your body but also your spirit, giving yourself the best foundation for a beautiful, balanced life. Remember, wellness isn't a destination; it's a journey. And every step you take toward connecting with yourself is a step toward a healthier, happier you.

When we give a little attention to the connection between our bodies and minds, we're not just improving our mood—we're boosting our health. A balanced nervous, endocrine, and immune system isn't just about feeling good; it's about creating a solid foundation for health, wellness, and beauty. Think of these practices as investments in your well-being. Each deep breath, each moment of laughter, and each step you take to nurture yourself is a gift to both your mind and body.

So, next time life throws a challenge your way, remember: you've got an internal team of messengers and systems working to keep you grounded, strong, and resilient. Nurture them, and they'll nurture you right back. And hey, who doesn't want a reason to laugh, breathe, and enjoy a little extra chocolate?

CHAPTER 9
ENERGY HEALING
UNLOCK YOUR BODY'S NATURAL HEALING ENERGY FOR RADIANCE AND VITALITY

In our high-speed, modern lives, we often dismiss the invisible forces that sustain and connect us. But for centuries, cultures around the world have recognized something profound: we are not just flesh and bone. We are also energetic beings, radiating and interacting with a field of energy that binds our body, mind, and spirit together. This field, often referred to as the "biofield," is the foundation of energy healing —a practice that can bring balance, calm, and even vitality into our lives.

WHAT IS THE BIOFIELD?

Think of the biofield as your body's personal Wi-Fi network— an invisible but essential system that keeps everything connected and functioning smoothly. This field surrounds and flows through your body, acting as an energetic bridge between your mind, body, and environment. It carries and responds to information from various sources, including physical, emotional, and mental influences.

1. **Electrical Energy:** Think about your heart beating or your brain sending signals to your muscles—these are electrical impulses that your body constantly

generates. Your biofield reflects and interacts with these natural electrical signals.

2. **Magnetic Energy:** Every time your heart beats, it creates a magnetic field. This isn't something you can see, but science has shown that the heart's magnetic field can extend several feet beyond the body. Your biofield interacts with these magnetic patterns, influencing your overall energy.

3. **Electromagnetic Energy:** This refers to the combination of electrical and magnetic energy. For example, the energy created by your body's cells working together, or even how your body responds to external sources like sunlight or the electromagnetic fields from electronic devices.

4. **Emotions and Thoughts:** Here's where it gets really personal. When you feel emotions like joy, love, or stress, or when you think positive or negative thoughts, these also create energetic ripples. Your biofield picks up on these vibrations, reflecting your internal state. For instance, prolonged negative emotions can disrupt this field, while feelings of gratitude or calm can harmonize it.

Think of it this way: just as music is a combination of sound waves creating harmony or dissonance, your biofield is shaped by the "notes" of your body's physical processes and your emotional and mental state. When everything is in balance, you're in tune—feeling good and vibrant. When it's out of balance, it's like your energy is playing a discordant tune, which can affect your well-being.

REAL-LIFE EXAMPLE

Have you ever met someone who instantly makes you feel calm and uplifted, as if their very presence soothes your stress? Or, on the flip side, someone whose energy leaves you feeling drained or tense? That's the interaction of biofields at play. Our biofields constantly communicate and respond to the energies around us, just like how a phone interacts with a Wi-Fi network.

Think of it like this: when you're in a crowded area, your phone might lose its signal due to interference. Similarly, your biofield can become "static" or disrupted when surrounded by conflicting or overwhelming energies. Keeping your biofield balanced is like maintaining a strong, clear signal—it allows you to stay centered, grounded, and connected to your inner peace, even in the midst of life's chaos.

THE BIOFIELD AND HEALING PRACTICES

In energy healing, many modalities—such as Reiki and Therapeutic Touch—aim to balance the biofield. You can think of these practices like a "tune-up" for your energy field, helping it function at its best. A simple example is when someone rubs their hands together before placing them on an area of pain or tension. The warmth and intention help balance the energy in that spot.

CHAKRAS AND MERIDIANS: THE HIGHWAYS OF ENERGY

Energy healing often focuses on the body's natural pathways, including chakras and meridians. You can think of chakras as energy hubs and meridians as highways that connect these hubs throughout your body.

Chakras: Your Energy Hubs

The concept of chakras comes from ancient Indian traditions, where they're seen as spinning wheels of energy located along the spine. Each chakra corresponds to different physical, emotional, and spiritual aspects.

The Solar Plexus Chakra (Located in the Upper Abdomen)

The Solar Plexus Chakra, also called the Manipura Chakra, is often referred to as the "power center." It governs self-confidence, personal power, and self-esteem. When this chakra is balanced, you feel capable, confident, and resilient. When blocked, you might experience insecurity, low self-esteem, or even physical issues like digestive discomfort.

Imagine you're preparing for a big presentation or facing a challenging conversation. That flutter in your stomach or tight knot of tension? That's your Solar Plexus talking. To balance this chakra and regain your confidence, you can visualize a warm yellow light glowing in your upper abdomen.

Why Yellow Light?

Yellow is the color traditionally associated with the Solar Plexus Chakra. Here's why:

- **Energy and Vitality:** Yellow represents the energy of sunlight, radiating warmth and life. It symbolizes the personal energy stored in your Solar Plexus, empowering you to take action and pursue your goals.
- **Mental Clarity:** Just like sunlight illuminates and brightens the world, yellow light fosters clarity and focus. Visualizing it helps you center your thoughts and build inner strength.
- **Confidence and Positivity:** Yellow is a color of happiness, optimism, and resilience—qualities essential for strong self-esteem and personal power.
- **Frequency Alignment:** In ancient teachings, each chakra vibrates at a specific frequency, and yellow aligns with the Solar Plexus Chakra's frequency, making it the ideal color to work with during visualization.

By imagining this yellow light, you're essentially "tuning in" to the Solar Plexus Chakra's energy. Picture the light radiating outward, dissolving tension, and infusing you with confidence and clarity. It's like summoning the sun within you to illuminate your path and ground your sense of self.

Electrical Fields: Your Body's Natural Signals

Did you know that every heartbeat and brainwave sends out tiny electrical impulses? It's true—your body is constantly buzzing with electrical activity. In fact, devices like EKGs (electrocardiograms) and EEGs (electroencephalograms) can pick up on these signals to assess the health of your heart and brain.

Ever touched a metal surface and felt a mild shock? That's your body's electrical field reacting to a different charge. It's a small but fascinating reminder that we're electrically active beings, even if we don't always feel it.

Magnetic Fields: Invisible Yet Powerful

Your heart and brain don't just generate electrical fields; they also create magnetic fields. These fields are so real that they can be measured with advanced tools like MEG (magnetoencephalography) and MCG (magnetocardiography).

You might have unknowingly interacted with magnetic fields, too. For instance, some people wear magnetic bracelets for joint pain relief. While the science isn't fully settled, the idea is that these bracelets may interact with your body's natural magnetic field to promote balance and ease discomfort.

Meridians: The Body's Energy Highways

Think of meridians as your body's energy superhighways, connecting different parts of you. Traditional Chinese Medicine (TCM) identifies 12 main meridians, each linked to specific organs and functions. When energy flows freely along these pathways, you feel balanced and healthy. But when there's a blockage, it can manifest as physical discomfort or emotional stress.

Take the Liver Meridian, for example. This pathway is associated with emotions like frustration or anger. If you've ever felt irritable or tense, you might benefit from stimulating a point on this meridian. A simple tip: Give yourself a foot massage or press gently on the webbing between your big toe and second toe. It's a known Liver Meridian point, and activating it can help ease tension and restore a sense of calm.

ACUPUNCTURE AND ACUPRESSURE: UNLOCKING THE BODY'S ENERGY POINTS

You've probably heard of acupuncture, where tiny needles are used to stimulate specific points along the body's meridians. But did you know there's a needle-free alternative? Enter acupressure, where you use your fingers to press and massage these same energy points.

Both techniques share the same goal: to clear energy blockages and restore balance in the body. Think of it as clearing a traffic jam on your body's energy highways—it gets everything moving smoothly again.

Why try these practices? Because they've been shown to do wonders for both your physical and emotional well-being. From easing pain and reducing stress to improving digestion and giving your skin a healthy glow, acupuncture and acupressure are powerful tools in holistic health.

A quick at-home tip: Feeling a headache coming on? Gently press and massage the space between your thumb and index finger (a well-known acupressure point called LI-4). It's often referred to as the "anti-stress button" and can help relieve tension in minutes.

What Is Acupuncture and How Does It Work?

Acupuncture might sound like something out of a medieval knight's survival guide, but rest assured—it's far from scary. This ancient practice, rooted in Traditional Chinese Medicine (TCM), uses fine, sterile needles inserted into specific points on the body, known as acupoints. The goal? To stimulate the flow of energy, or Qi (pronounced "chee"), along the body's energy pathways called meridians.

Think of Qi as your body's Wi-Fi signal. When it's strong, everything runs smoothly—your mood is up, your digestion is on point, and your stress? Managed. But when the signal gets interrupted (thanks to stress, poor sleep, or life in general), that's when pain, tension, or health issues sneak in. Acupuncture works like a Wi-Fi extender for your energy, clearing blockages and getting your body back online.

Benefits of Acupuncture

Acupuncture isn't just an ancient mystery—it's gained modern-day street cred for addressing a wide range of issues. Here's what it can do for you:

- **Pain Relief:** Got a back that feels like it belongs to a 90-year-old or migraines that won't quit? Acupuncture stimulates the release of endorphins, your body's natural painkillers. Think of it as giving your pain a soothing "shush."
- **Stress Reduction:** Acupuncture helps regulate your nervous system, lowering stress and cortisol levels. It's like a spa day for your mind—without the hefty price tag.
- **Digestive Health:** Whether it's bloating, acid reflux, or a stomach that grumbles like it's auditioning for a horror movie, acupuncture supports energy flow through your digestive system for smoother operations.

- **Improved Sleep:** Counting sheep not working? Acupuncture can help calm your mind and regulate your body's sleep-wake cycle, giving you a ticket to dreamland.
- **Immune Support:** Regular acupuncture sessions can strengthen your immune system, making you feel like you're wearing an invisible superhero cape against colds and flu.
- **Chronic Illness Relief:** From fibromyalgia to allergies to infertility, acupuncture has been shown to provide relief by supporting your body's natural healing processes.

What Does It Feel Like?

If the word "needles" sends a shiver down your spine, relax! The needles used in acupuncture are so thin they make sewing needles look bulky. Most people describe the sensation as a slight tingling, warmth, or gentle pressure—definitely not the "ouch!" you might expect.

In fact, sessions are designed to be relaxing. Imagine lying down in a quiet room while someone works magic on your energy pathways. Many people report feeling calm and rejuvenated afterward, as if their body just took a much-needed vacation.

Acupuncture is essentially the "multi-tool" of health practices —whether you're tackling chronic pain, looking for better sleep, or just want to feel more balanced, it's worth considering. And let's be honest, who doesn't need a little extra balance in life?

How Acupressure Works

At my workplace, I've seen countless patients benefit from acupressure. It's a gentle yet powerful practice that anyone can do at home to balance energy, relieve pain, and support overall wellness. Unlike acupuncture, there are no needles involved—

just your fingers, thumbs, or even a smooth, rounded tool. Think of it as your body's very own DIY tune-up.

Acupressure works by releasing energy blockages that often manifest as pain or tension. And the best part? You don't need a medical degree to try it. With the right guidance, you can become your own energy healer, no white coat required.

Acupressure: A Hands-On Healing Practice

Performing acupressure on yourself is easier than you might think. It's essentially the art of giving your body some TLC (tender loving care)—but with a purpose. Let's break it down:

How to Perform Acupressure on Yourself

1. Find a Quiet Space

Start by finding a calm, comfortable spot where you won't be disturbed. Sit or lie down, take a few deep breaths, and tell your body, "Alright, let's fix this mess!"

2. Locate the Pressure Point

Use a guide (like this chapter) to locate the acupressure point. Don't worry if it feels a bit like playing "pin the tail on the donkey" at first—it gets easier with practice.

3. Apply Gentle, Firm Pressure

Apply pressure firmly but gently, like you're pressing a button on an old TV remote. You should feel a slight tenderness, but it shouldn't hurt. (If it does, your body's saying, "Hey, ease up!")

4. Breathe and Focus

As you hold the point, take deep breaths and imagine tension melting away like ice cream on a hot day. And if your mind wanders to what's for dinner, that's okay—just gently bring your focus back.

A Quick Example: The Famous "Liver Meridian Point"

Feeling irritable or stressed? Try pressing on the webbing between your big toe and the second toe (a point along the Liver Meridian). It's like a reset button for built-up frustration. And hey, it doubles as a sneaky way to give yourself a mini foot massage!

Do's and Don'ts of Acupressure

Getting the most out of acupressure is all about balance—literally and figuratively. Here are some simple guidelines to help you practice safely and effectively:

Do's

- Apply steady, even pressure, and pair it with mindful, deep breathing to amplify the calming effects.
- Listen to your body—if a point feels tender or too sensitive, ease up on the pressure. It's about relief, not discomfort.

Don'ts

- Avoid pressing on bruised, swollen, or broken skin. Acupressure is about healing, not adding to the problem.
- Skip acupressure immediately after a heavy meal. Give your digestion a chance to work its magic without interruptions.

Frequency and Duration

Consistency is key, but don't stress about perfection. Aim to perform acupressure once or twice a day on areas that need attention. Sessions typically last 5-10 minutes, but listen to your body—if a spot feels sore, take a break and give it some love later.

Morning sessions are fantastic for an energizing start, while evening sessions can help you unwind. Find what fits into your rhythm, whether it's during your morning coffee ritual or as part of your bedtime wind-down routine.

Specific Acupressure Points for Common Concerns

Here's a quick guide to some go-to points you can use to tackle everyday challenges:

Anxiety Relief (Pericardium 6)

- **Where to find it:** Three finger-widths below your wrist, between two tendons.
- **Why it works:** Pressing this point can help ease anxiety and reduce nausea.
- **How to do it:** Apply gentle pressure for 1-2 minutes whenever you're feeling overwhelmed—think of it as your personal "reset button."

Headache Relief (LI4)

- **Where to find it:** The fleshy spot between your thumb and index finger.
- **Why it works:** This point is a classic for relieving tension headaches and migraines.
- **How to do it:** Use firm, circular pressure for 1-2 minutes on each hand. Bonus tip: Start pressing when you feel the first signs of a headache—it can work wonders!

Energy Boost (Stomach 36)

- **Where to find it:** Four finger-widths below your kneecap.

- **Why it works:** This point is like a shot of espresso for your body, boosting energy and aiding digestion.
- **How to do it:** Press it in the morning for a steady stream of vitality throughout the day.

Beauty and Skin Glow (Stomach 3)

- **Where to find it:** Right under your cheekbones.
- **Why it works:** Stimulating this point improves circulation to your face, reducing puffiness and giving your skin a natural glow.
- **How to do it:** Use gentle, circular pressure for a minute or two as part of your skincare routine. Glow, baby, glow!

Hair Health (GV20)

- **Where to find it:** The very top of your head (imagine balancing a book there).
- **Why it works:** Massaging this point encourages blood flow to your scalp, which can support hair growth.
- **How to do it:** Gently massage the area for 1-2 minutes daily. It's like a mini scalp spa session!By integrating these acupressure points into your routine, you're giving your body the tools to restore balance and thrive. Whether it's calming your mind, tackling headaches, or adding that extra glow to your beauty routine, acupressure is your accessible, go-anywhere wellness companion.

By integrating these acupressure points into your routine, you're giving your body the tools to restore balance and thrive. Whether it's calming your mind, tackling headaches, or adding that extra glow to your beauty routine, acupressure is your accessible, go-anywhere wellness companion.

EMBRACING ENERGY HEALING IN DAILY LIFE

Energy healing isn't about lengthy rituals or fancy tools—it's about weaving small, intentional practices into your routine to harmonize your body and mind.

By tuning into your biofield, balancing your chakras, and practicing acupressure on key points, you're essentially giving yourself a daily recharge. It's like plugging your inner battery into a power source that leaves you feeling grounded, vital, and beautifully balanced.

Think of these techniques as your personal wellness toolkit. Whether it's a moment of deep breathing during a chaotic day, visualizing that yellow light for confidence, or gently pressing acupressure points for relief, every small act adds up.

These practices aren't just about healing; they're about thriving—helping you face life's challenges with clarity, calm, and a glow that radiates from the inside out.

CONCLUSION: HARNESSING THE POWER WITHIN

Energy healing is more than just a practice—it's a journey back to yourself. By understanding and nurturing the intricate connection between your body, mind, and energy, you can unlock a wellspring of calm, vitality, and inner beauty. Each intentional breath, gentle press on an acupressure point, or visualization of light is a step toward harmony—a gift you give yourself in a world that often demands so much.

Remember, your energy is your greatest asset. When you take the time to balance it, you're not only improving your health and well-being but also showing up in the world as your most vibrant, confident self. Energy healing empowers you to take control of how you feel, look, and move through life.

YOUR CALL TO ACTION

Start today. Choose one practice from this chapter—whether it's mindful breathing, acupressure, or visualizing a glowing yellow light—and make it part of your routine. Just five minutes a day can create a ripple effect, transforming how you feel inside and radiating outward.

You don't need to be an expert. You only need the willingness to try. Trust the process, and watch as these small acts of self-care unlock your inner power, bringing balance, resilience, and undeniable radiance into your life.

You hold the key to your energy—now go unlock it!

CHAPTER 10
FIGHTING COLDS, KEEPING YOUR GLOW
HEALTH AND BEAUTY ESSENTIALS

 "Our bodies are our gardens—our wills are our gardeners."

— William Shakespeare

As a mother, one of my most essential duties is ensuring my whole family stays healthy. Unfortunately, little kids are prone to getting sick easily and often.

When I had my first child, I followed the old adage that the common cold was just part of life. I thought isolating him from the playground and letting him rest would be enough. But as his cold worsened, I grew more concerned. Eventually, I took him to the doctor, who told me there wasn't much to be done since colds are viral. He advised me to make sure my son rested and stayed hydrated.

Despite this advice, his condition deteriorated. He began coughing so hard that it terrified me. I finally took him to urgent care, where he was diagnosed with pneumonia. It was a terrifying and stressful experience for all of us.

Since that day, I've become far more proactive about managing illnesses from the very beginning. I've learned the importance of preventative measures to naturally boost the immune system, keeping it strong enough to fight future sickness. I've made it my mission to ensure my children eat a balanced diet with nutritious foods from all categories: fruits, vegetables, carbohydrates, and proteins.

Of course, getting kids to eat all these foods isn't always easy. That's why I also rely on high-quality liquid vitamin supplements for better absorption. At the first sign of a runny nose or cough, I take immediate, aggressive steps to provide my children with the nourishment they need.

My go-to remedies include honey-lemon drinks—a natural immunity booster—along with probiotics like yogurt and soothing chicken soup. I explain to my kids that our bodies have two kinds of germs: the good and the bad. The good germs act as our body's soldiers, fighting off the bad ones. By eating nutritious foods, we make our soldiers stronger, giving them the power to protect us from illness.

This simple analogy resonates with them, and I believe it's a concept we all can embrace in our daily lives. Supporting our body's natural defenses can significantly reduce the frequency and severity of the illnesses we face.

In this chapter, we'll explore what the common cold and flu are, how they affect both our health and appearance, and effective strategies to prevent and manage them while maintaining your glow.

WHAT ARE THE COMMON COLD AND FLU?

Let's break it down: both the common cold and the flu are respiratory illnesses, but they're caused by different viruses and have their own personalities. The flu, brought on by the influenza virus, tends to hit hard and fast—it's like an uninvited guest who storms in, makes a mess, and leaves you feeling wiped out. The common cold, on the other hand, is caused by over 200 different viruses. It's less dramatic, but it can linger, poking at you with mild symptoms that disrupt your day.

So, why is the flu often worse even though it stems from just one virus? Think of it this way: the flu is like a single villain in a blockbuster movie—it's focused, powerful, and determined to take center stage. The common cold, with its hundreds of viruses, is more like a crowd of minor troublemakers. Individually, they're less intense, but they can still leave you feeling off balance if you're not careful.

HOW TO TELL THE DIFFERENCE: SYMPTOMS OF COLD VS. FLU

- **Flu Symptoms**:
  - Sudden onset of fever and chills
  - Body aches and fatigue (the kind that makes you want to live in your bed)
  - Dry cough and sore throat
  - Headaches
  - Occasionally nausea or diarrhea (especially in kids)
- **Cold Symptoms**:
  - Runny or stuffy nose
  - Sneezing
  - Mild cough
  - Scratchy throat
  - Sometimes a low-grade fever

Here's the good news: While the flu demands a lot more attention and care (and sometimes a trip to the doctor), the common cold usually runs its course with a little rest, hydration, and self-care. But don't take either lightly—your health deserves priority, even if it's "just a cold."

A RELATABLE TAKE FOR WOMEN

Picture this: The flu is like a toddler having a full-blown tantrum in the middle of the grocery store—loud, disruptive, and hard to ignore. The common cold? It's like a persistent friend who texts you nonstop—it's not as intense, but it still gets on your nerves. Both demand your attention, but the key is knowing how to respond without letting them steal your glow.

Take it from me: whether it's a cold or the flu, your body is calling for care and attention. Listen to it, nurture it, and remember—this too shall pass (and you'll look fabulous on the other side).

THE HIDDEN TOLL OF COMMON ILLNESSES ON HEALTH AND APPEARANCE

Let's face it—when you're sick, you don't just feel awful; you look it too. It's rare to see someone battling a cold or flu who also radiates joy and vitality. Sickness takes a toll on your body, mood, and yes, your appearance. The common cold and flu aren't just minor inconveniences—they can leave a lasting impact on your health and how you present yourself to the world.

While most people recover from a cold or flu within a week or two, those with weakened immune systems can experience longer bouts of illness. Fatigue, dehydration, and muscle aches become constant companions, and in severe cases, the flu can lead to more dangerous complications like pneumonia. These viruses don't just attack your energy levels—they can wreak havoc on your skin too.

HOW ILLNESS IMPACTS YOUR SKIN

Let's not sugarcoat it: colds and the flu have a knack for amplifying your worst skin days. The constant nose-blowing? It leaves your skin red, chapped, and irritated. The dehydration that comes with fever? It sucks the moisture out of your skin, leaving it dull and flaky. And those dark circles under your eyes? They're practically shouting to the world, "I haven't slept in days!"

Dry skin, fine lines, and wrinkles can appear more pronounced when your body is dehydrated. Cracked lips and irritated hands and feet add to the misery, making it feel like your entire body is crying out for relief.

SELF-CARE FOR YOUR SKIN DURING COLD AND FLU SEASON: A WOMAN'S GUIDE

Ladies, let's be honest—when we're under the weather, juggling the responsibilities of life with looking and feeling good feels nearly impossible. But don't worry, I've got your back. Here are some quick and easy beauty and skincare tips to keep you glowing even on your worst days.

Quick Beauty and Wellness Boosters for Sick Days

Being under the weather doesn't mean you have to feel—or look—completely run down. These simple beauty and self-care tips will help you combat the visible effects of colds and flu while giving you a much-needed confidence boost.

Puffy Eyes? Say Goodbye

Tired, puffy eyes are a dead giveaway that you're sick. Fight back with a quick DIY treatment: brew a comforting cup of black tea, then chill the tea bags and place them over your eyes for 10-15 minutes. The caffeine constricts blood vessels, and the cold reduces swelling—leaving you looking refreshed and less congested. Plus, it's the perfect excuse to sit back and relax.

Soothe Chapped and Irritated Skin

A red, sore nose is no fun, but it's manageable. Opt for moisturizers with soothing ingredients like hyaluronic acid, aloe vera, or coconut oil to calm irritated skin and lock in hydration. A dab of Vaseline around your nose and lips can work wonders, too, especially when the skin feels extra raw. Bonus: these same remedies double as lifesavers for cracked hands and heels.

Hydrate Those Lips and More

Dry, chapped lips are another unwelcome side effect of illness. Start with the basics: drink plenty of water throughout the day, especially before bed. Skip dehydrating culprits like salty snacks, coffee, and (yes, brace yourself) wine. And, of course, keep a trusty lip balm nearby for quick relief.

Humidifiers: Your Secret Weapon

If you don't have a humidifier yet, now's the time to invest in one. Humidifiers add moisture to the air, which is a game-changer for your skin and sinuses. Not only will it help you breathe easier at night, but it will also prevent that dreaded "desert-dry" skin. Think of it as a spa treatment for your face while you sleep—wake up with smoother skin and clearer nasal passages. It's a win-win!

Keep Hydration a Priority

Staying hydrated isn't just about drinking water. Incorporate water-rich foods like cucumbers, oranges, and watermelon into your meals. Fresh juices, such as carrot or green juice, can give you a nutrient boost—just dilute them if you're watching your sugar intake. Hydration helps your body recover faster and keeps your skin plump and glowing, even during sick days.

Rest is Your Best Beauty Remedy

Finally, don't underestimate the power of good sleep. Rest is when your body repairs itself, from your skin to your immune system. If congestion keeps you tossing and turning, prop your pillows up to ease breathing and let your humidifier work its magic. The result? A more refreshed, glowing you.

GOING THE EXTRA MILE FOR YOUR SKIN

Inhale, Exhale, Refresh

When your skin looks as tired as you feel and congestion has you down, steam inhalation is your at-home rescue. Here's how: boil some water, pour it into a large bowl, and lean over it with a towel draped over your head. For an extra boost, add a few drops of essential oils like eucalyptus or tea tree. Not only will these oils help clear your airways, but their antioxidants and anti-inflammatory properties will give your skin a rejuvenating boost. Think of it as a mini facial and a breathing treatment rolled into one. Your sinuses will thank you, and so will your complexion.

You Are What You Eat: Nourish to Flourish

It's easy to overlook nutrition when you're under the weather, but what you put into your body directly affects how you look and feel. Nutrient-rich foods are your secret weapon. Vitamins A, C, and E, along with antioxidant-packed options like oranges and blueberries, do double duty: strengthening your immune system and giving your skin a glow from the inside out.

Picture this: while you're munching on a handful of nuts or savoring a colorful smoothie, you're not just satisfying hunger—you're building an army of internal defenders and nourishing your skin at the same time. It's like sending a heartfelt care package to your body, reminding yourself that you're loved, even on the hardest days. Go ahead, indulge in self-care through food—your immune system and complexion will thank you.

CONQUER THE COMMON COLD: A WOMAN'S GUIDE TO IMMUNITY AND WELLNESS

Let's face it: life doesn't stop when a cold hits. Whether you're a parent juggling caregiving duties or a professional balancing work and home, colds don't discriminate. According to WebMD, adults average 2 to 4 colds a year, and as women, we're often the ones nurturing everyone else back to health—leaving ourselves exposed to all those germs.

But are we just going to let a pesky cold slow us down? Absolutely not.

Here's the deal: our bodies are incredible. They're like fortresses, equipped with warrior-like immune cells ready to fend off invaders. But fortresses need upkeep. A strong immune system starts with hydration, nutrition, and self-care. With a little intention and the right tools, we can keep the drawbridge up and the viruses out.

So here's your rallying cry: life's too vibrant and full of opportunities to let a common cold sideline you. We're strong, resilient women—capable of managing households, thriving in careers, and building our dreams. A cold? That's just a minor detour, not a roadblock. Let's fortify ourselves and reclaim our health, one small, intentional step at a time.

UPPER RESPIRATORY INFECTIONS: MY FAMILY'S APPROACH TO NATURAL REMEDIES

In my family, upper respiratory infections (URIs)—a.k.a. the dreaded common cold—are like that annoying guest who shows up uninvited and overstays their welcome. Over the years, I've taken on the role of natural remedies detective, experimenting with herbs and supplements to boost our immune systems and send those pesky colds packing.

After plenty of trial and error (and a few "oops, maybe that wasn't the right herb" moments), I've curated a list of cold-fighting staples that have become permanent fixtures in our home. Let me introduce you to our go-to lineup and the science behind their magic:

Echinacea: The Immune System's Superhero

Echinacea is packed with compounds like **phenols** and **alkamides**, which have antioxidant and anti-inflammatory properties. Phenols help protect cells from free radical damage, while alkamides work to enhance the activity of immune cells. This combination makes echinacea a go-to for reducing cold symptoms and boosting overall immunity.

Pro Tip: Timing is crucial. Start taking echinacea at the first sign of a sniffle for the best results. And if you have an autoimmune condition, consult a healthcare provider first—it may not be the best choice for you.

Astragalus: The Ancient Warrior

Astragalus is a staple in Traditional Chinese Medicine and earns its spot with components like **polysaccharides**, **saponins**, and **flavonoids**.

- **Polysaccharides** enhance the body's ability to fight infections by boosting the activity of white blood cells.
- **Saponins** are known for their anti-inflammatory and immune-regulating properties.
- **Flavonoids** act as antioxidants, protecting your cells from damage caused by oxidative stress.

While more modern research is needed, these components make astragalus a trusted choice for building long-term immunity and keeping seasonal illnesses at bay.

Elderberry: The Cold-Fighting Ninja

Elderberries are rich in **anthocyanins**, the pigments responsible for their deep purple color and powerful antioxidant properties. Anthocyanins help reduce inflammation and boost cytokine production, which supports the immune system in fighting off viruses.

- **Vitamin C and dietary fiber** in elderberries also contribute to their immune-boosting effects.
- Elderberry has been shown in studies to reduce the severity and duration of colds and flu, making it a family favorite in syrup or lozenge form.

Pro Tip: Elderberry syrup tastes amazing, making it a hit with kids—and adults won't mind taking it either!

Vitamin C: The Immunity Booster

Vitamin C, or ascorbic acid, is a powerhouse antioxidant that supports various cellular functions of the immune system.

- It helps stimulate the production of **white blood cells**, which are crucial for defending against infections.
- Vitamin C also strengthens the skin's barrier function, acting as a physical shield against pathogens.

Aim for **500 to 1000 mg daily** during cold and flu season to keep your immune system ready for battle.

Zinc: The Cellular Repair Specialist

Zinc is a trace mineral that plays a vital role in immune defense by supporting the activity of over 300 enzymes in the body.

- It helps regulate **inflammatory responses** and activates certain immune cells, such as T-cells.
- Zinc also has direct antiviral properties, making it especially effective when taken within **24 hours of the onset of symptoms**.

Stick to **75 to 100 mg per day** to maximize its cold-shortening benefits, but be careful not to overdo it, as excessive zinc can interfere with the absorption of other essential minerals.

SHOPPING SMART: QUALITY MATTERS

When it comes to buying supplements, not all products are created equal. Look for ones that are **third-party tested** to ensure quality and avoid unnecessary additives. After all, if you're going to invest in your health, it's worth knowing exactly what you're putting into your body.

By understanding what makes each herb and supplement effective, you'll not only feel more confident in your choices but also be better equipped to share this knowledge with your loved ones. So, stock up on these immune-boosting allies and keep your family healthy and glowing, even during cold and flu season!

QUICK FIXES TO EASE SYMPTOMS: SALT WATER GARGLES

Ever wondered why your grandma swore by salt water gargles for a sore throat? Turns out, she was onto something—and there's solid science to back it up. Let's break it down in a way that'll make you appreciate this humble remedy even more:

- **A Mini Spa for Your Throat:** Gargling with salt water acts like a soothing massage for those irritated throat cells. The salt gently draws out excess water from swollen tissues, reducing inflammation and that raw, scratchy feeling. It's like hitting the pause button on throat discomfort.
- **Bacteria's Worst Host:** While salt doesn't kill bacteria outright, it does create an environment that's far from cozy for them. Think of it as dimming the lights and turning off the music at a party—the unwelcome guests (aka germs) will get the hint and leave.
- **Clearing Out Mucus:** Sticky mucus clogging your throat? Salt water gargles help loosen that goo, making it easier to swallow and breathe. It's like clearing a blocked hallway so everything flows smoothly again.
- **Warmth for Instant Comfort:** There's something undeniably comforting about warm salt water. It's like wrapping your sore throat in a soft, cozy blanket—instantly soothing and oh-so-calming.
- **Hydration Helper:** Just like your favorite houseplants thrive with the right amount of water,

your throat needs moisture to heal. Gargling helps keep things hydrated, preventing further irritation and dryness.

So, the next time your throat feels like sandpaper, channel your inner grandma and reach for a mug of warm salt water. It's simple, effective, and comforting—a tried-and-true remedy that stands the test of time.

Pro Tip: While this remedy works wonders for mild discomfort, don't hesitate to call your doctor if the soreness lingers or worsens. Think of them as the ultimate backup singers for your throat's solo performance!

GARGLING WITH DILUTED LISTERINE: A REFRESHING TWIST FOR THROAT CARE

When throat discomfort strikes, a simple remedy might be closer than you think—right in your bathroom cabinet! Gargling with **diluted Listerine mouthwash** is a modern, refreshing way to ease a sore throat.

Why Listerine? Known for its powerful antiseptic properties, this household staple is designed to combat oral bacteria, and when diluted, it can extend its cleansing magic to your throat. The key here is **dilution**—think of it as mellowing your coffee with cream to avoid the "too strong" effect. Using undiluted Listerine can be harsh, but a little water transforms it into a soothing solution for mild irritation.

Plus, it leaves your mouth feeling minty fresh—a bonus when you're not exactly feeling your best. Just remember, if your symptoms persist, always consult a healthcare professional to make sure there's nothing more serious going on.

APPLE CIDER VINEGAR GARGLE: A ZESTY DEFENSE FOR YOUR THROAT

Feeling that telltale scratchiness in your throat? It might be time to give **apple cider vinegar** a try. This tangy remedy blends traditional wisdom with modern wellness and is as simple as mixing vinegar with water for a gentle gargle.

Why does it work? Apple cider vinegar is celebrated for its natural antibacterial properties, making it a gentle defender against throat irritants. Its slightly acidic nature can also help break down mucus, providing relief from that tight, scratchy feeling.

What makes this remedy stand out is the **zesty experience**—the tangy flavor can be surprisingly invigorating, offering a pick-me-up for your senses while helping your throat feel better. It's perfect for those who enjoy an unconventional yet effective health hack.

Pro Tip: Always dilute apple cider vinegar before using it as a gargle to keep it gentle on your throat. And if your discomfort lingers, don't hesitate to reach out to a healthcare professional.

COMFORT IN A CUP: DRINKS THAT HEAL AND SOOTHE

Imagine this: the sky outside is heavy with gray clouds, and the chill in the air invites you to slow down. You're wrapped in your coziest blanket, your favorite book in one hand, and in the other? A steaming mug of wellness magic—your secret weapon against the common cold.

Hot Honey Lemonade: Your Cozy Defense

This isn't just a drink; it's a hug in a cup. Honey doesn't just sweeten—it works wonders for soothing irritated throats. Its antimicrobial properties are like a gentle army, fighting off those pesky germs that are overstaying their welcome. Lemon, on the other hand, is your dose of liquid sunshine, packed with

Vitamin C to give your immune system a much-needed boost. Together, they're like the dream team your body needs during cold season.

But there's more to this classic than science. Each sip is a reminder of simpler times—maybe a loved one brewing this comforting concoction when you were feeling under the weather. It's more than hydration; it's a moment of self-care, one that warms both body and soul.

Pro Tip: Add a pinch of ginger for an extra kick of anti-inflammatory goodness. It'll not only amp up the flavor but also help reduce any lingering aches.

The Citrus Elixir: A Zesty Revival

For those days when your cold feels like it's taken control, meet the apple cider vinegar citrus elixir. This vibrant blend of apple cider vinegar, orange juice, lemon juice, and a pinch of pink salt is like an energy boost for your immune system.

- **Apple Cider Vinegar**: Known for its antibacterial properties, it's the wise old sage of home remedies, helping to create a less hospitable environment for germs.
- **Citrus Power**: The orange and lemon juices aren't just for zest; they're packed with Vitamin C, which helps reduce the severity and duration of colds by supporting your immune system's front lines.
- **Pink Salt**: Adding a whisper of minerals and electrolytes, it helps balance the bold flavors and keeps you hydrated when your body is fighting off illness.

Every sip feels like a tiny celebration for your body, blending tartness with a subtle warmth that feels just right. It's not just a drink—it's a moment to pause and nourish yourself, even when you're feeling less than your best.

WHY THESE DRINKS WORK: THE SCIENCE OF SIPPING WELLNESS

- **Hydration**: Fighting a cold depletes your body's fluids. Warm drinks help keep you hydrated while soothing your throat and loosening mucus.
- **Immune Boosting**: The Vitamin C in citrus fruits helps reduce cold symptoms and supports faster recovery. Honey's antimicrobial properties offer additional support.
- **Soothing Warmth**: The heat from these drinks can relax your throat, reduce congestion, and provide comfort that feels like a spa day for your insides.

A Sip of Comfort, A Moment of Care

The next time a cold tries to bring you down, remember: these simple, natural drinks are your allies. Whether it's the sweet embrace of hot honey lemonade or the invigorating zest of a citrus elixir, you're not just treating symptoms—you're showing yourself a little love. And isn't that what wellness is all about?

Now, go grab your favorite mug, wrap yourself in that blanket, and savor every sip. You've got this, one comforting gulp at a time.

THE HEALING EMBRACE OF CHICKEN SOUP: MORE THAN COMFORT FOOD

Ah, chicken soup—the timeless remedy that warms you from the inside out. It's not just a dish; it's a heartfelt tradition, a culinary hug in a bowl that generations have turned to during cold and flu season. But did you know there's actual science behind its healing powers? This humble broth does more than soothe your soul; it supports your body in surprising ways.

A Natural Decongestant

Ever noticed how steam rising from a hot bowl of chicken soup seems to clear your stuffy nose? That's no coincidence. The warm vapor helps open nasal passages, making it easier to breathe. The soup's ingredients—garlic, onions, and herbs—often have mild anti-inflammatory properties, further aiding in reducing nasal congestion. Think of it as a gentle, natural decongestant working in harmony with your body.

Packed with Nutrients

Chicken soup isn't just comfort food—it's a nutrient-rich elixir. The broth, simmered with chicken bones, releases minerals like calcium, magnesium, and phosphorus, while the vegetables provide a hearty dose of vitamins. Carrots bring beta-carotene for immune support, celery aids hydration, and onions contribute quercetin, a natural anti-inflammatory compound. Together, they form a team of nourishing superheroes, helping to fortify your immune system when it needs it most.

Soothing for Sore Throats and Body Aches

There's something about the warmth of chicken soup that feels like a balm for a sore throat or tired body. The hot liquid coats your throat, alleviating irritation, while the protein-packed chicken offers amino acids like cysteine, which help thin mucus and make it easier to expel. It's like a tailored remedy, designed to ease your symptoms and give your body the comfort it craves.

Emotional Nourishment

Beyond the physical benefits, chicken soup holds an unparalleled emotional connection. It's often a dish lovingly made by someone who cares—your mom, grandma, or even yourself during self-care moments. Every spoonful can evoke a sense of nostalgia, of being cared for and nurtured. This emotional comfort plays a role in recovery, as feeling supported and calm is just as important as any medicine.

A Simple Yet Powerful Remedy

In today's world of over-the-counter quick fixes, chicken soup stands out as a reminder of the power of wholesome, traditional remedies. It's a beautiful blend of simplicity and effectiveness, proving that sometimes the best solutions don't come from a bottle but from a simmering pot in your kitchen.

So, when a cold has you feeling down, let chicken soup be your go-to remedy. It's more than a meal—it's a gentle embrace for your body, a comforting ritual for your mind, and a timeless gift for your spirit. One spoonful at a time, you'll feel a little better, inside and out.

YOUR INTERNAL ARMORY: SUPERFOODS THAT PACK A PUNCH

When it comes to keeping your immune system in top shape, certain foods are like your internal knights in shining armor. Spinach, ginger, and citrus fruits are more than just meal staples—they're the nutrient powerhouses your immune cells need to fight off invaders. Think of them as your secret weapon in the battle against colds and flu. Toss them into a smoothie, sauté them with dinner, or snack on them throughout the day. Your immune system will thank you!

YOUR CULINARY SHIELD: SPICES THAT HEAL

Garlic, onion, basil, and thyme aren't just flavor enhancers—they're nature's immune-boosting marvels. Garlic, for instance, contains allicin, which can help fend off infections. Basil and thyme are loaded with antioxidants to give your immune system that extra edge. So go ahead, sprinkle some of these culinary champions into your meals. They're like tiny shields of protection on your plate.

FIRST LINE OF DEFENSE: CLEAN HANDS, CLEAN LIFE

Handwashing is your front-line defense—your immune system's first knight. And don't stop there! Think about all those high-touch items like your phone, doorknobs, and remote controls. Keeping them clean can drastically reduce the chances of germs finding their way into your system. Make cleanliness a ritual—it's simple but oh-so-powerful.

THE SECRET WEAPON: SUPPLEMENT SMARTER

Supplements are like the underground tunnels that fortify your immune fortress—subtle but essential. My go-to immunity booster mix? Echinacea, astragalus, elderberry, vitamin C, and zinc. These gems work behind the scenes to strengthen your defenses and help you recover faster when illness strikes.

But remember, not all supplements are created equal. Always choose high-quality, third-party-tested options and consult your healthcare provider to ensure they're the right fit for your unique needs. Supplements aren't a cure-all, but when used wisely, they're an invaluable secret weapon for your health.

THE POWER OF EARLY INTERVENTION: LISTEN TO YOUR BODY

Ladies, let me tell you, your body is smarter than you think. It's like your best friend—it always sends you little hints when something's not quite right. Maybe it's a scratchy throat, low energy that has you dragging your fabulous self through the day, or just that off feeling you can't quite put your finger on. These are your body's gentle SOS signals saying, "Hey, pay attention to me!"

From my personal playbook, the moment my throat starts auditioning for the role of "villain in a scratchy horror movie," I know it's time to hit pause. Life can wait for a bit—it's time for some TLC.

First, I grab my go-to remedies. Gargling with apple cider vinegar mixed with warm salt water? Yes, it's as unglamorous as it sounds, but let me tell you—it's like a disinfectant for your throat, courtesy of Mother Nature. Then, I whip up hot, peppery soups (extra garlic for good measure—because garlic is life).

Next, I bring out my feel-good staples: honey-lemon drinks for that soothing hug in a mug, fragrant lemongrass teas to calm my nerves, and my trusty elderberry and echinacea supplements. These aren't just about pampering myself—there's science behind their magic. Honey is antibacterial, lemon is loaded with vitamin C, garlic boosts your immunity, and elderberry? It's like a ninja for cold and flu relief.

The lesson? Don't wait for your body to scream—listen when it whispers. Acting quickly can turn those tiny warning signs into a full-blown wellness win. So, next time your body sends out a signal, answer it like the queen you are and give it the care it deserves. Your future self will thank you.

IN SUMMARY: HONOR YOUR BODY, BUILD YOUR IMMUNITY FORTRESS

Ladies, here's the bottom line: your body is your greatest ally, and every little ache, scratch, or sniffle is its way of speaking to you. Don't dismiss those signals; honor them. Think of your immune system as a fortress—strong, resilient, and ready to protect you, but only if you provide the right tools and care.

Fortifying your immunity isn't just about dodging the common cold or flu; it's about creating a lifestyle where health, energy, and vibrance are your daily companions. It's about nourishing your body, listening to its whispers before they become shouts, and treating every moment of self-care as an act of love and empowerment.

You have the power to take control of your health journey.

Start small but stay consistent—drink your water, savor your soups, stock up on superfoods, and take that extra five minutes to rest when your body asks for it. Because thriving isn't just about avoiding illness; it's about living fully, glowing with vitality, and enjoying all the beautiful, messy, wonderful things life has to offer.

So, the next time you feel the faintest tickle in your throat or the slightest fatigue in your body, don't wait. Act swiftly, arm yourself with knowledge, and give your immune system the care it deserves. You're not just protecting yourself from a cold —you're setting the foundation for a stronger, healthier, and more radiant you.

Take the reins, build your fortress, and go live your incredible life to the fullest, because you deserve nothing less.

CHAPTER 11

THRIVING WITH DIABETES

YOUR GUIDE TO HEALTH, VITALITY, AND EMPOWERMENT

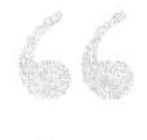 "The doctor of the future will give no medicine, but will involve the patient in the proper use of food, fresh air, and exercise."

— Thomas Edison

After fortifying our defenses against common illnesses in the previous chapter, let's turn our attention to a condition that demands lifelong vigilance: diabetes. This silent yet impactful challenge affects millions worldwide, and managing it effectively can mean the difference between merely surviving and truly thriving.

For me, diabetes hits close to home. As someone who has reviewed countless medical charts for diabetic patients, I also live its daily realities through my husband, who relies on insulin injections. It's not just about managing numbers on a chart—it's the emotional weight of seeing him sneak sugary treats or make choices he knows he shouldn't. If you've ever watched a loved one make decisions that scare you, you'll understand the tension and helplessness that can bring.

I'll admit, I used to play the role of "diet police," micromanaging his every meal to keep his condition in check. But that approach? It backfired spectacularly. He rebelled, the tension between us grew, and I found myself physically and emotionally drained. My sleep suffered, my mood soured, and even my skin bore the marks of stress.

Then, a moment of clarity changed everything. Real support doesn't come from nagging or controlling—it comes from love, understanding, and respect. Instead of policing his choices, I pivoted to becoming a cheerleader. I started cooking meals we could both enjoy, suggesting fun ways to stay active, and offering calm encouragement rather than criticism.

It's not easy to watch someone you care about make choices that worry you. But maintaining a supportive and empathetic mindset can reduce stress for everyone involved—including you.

If you or a loved one are managing diabetes, take heart. This chapter is your guide to proactive steps for not only managing the condition but also preserving your overall health and vibrance. Before we dive into actionable strategies, let's first unpack what diabetes is and how it impacts your well-being.

WHAT IS DIABETES?

Diabetes is a medical condition that interferes with the body's ability to properly use or store glucose, a type of sugar. There are two main culprits behind this dysfunction. In Type 2 diabetes, either the pancreas doesn't produce enough insulin, or the body develops what's known as "insulin resistance," meaning it doesn't use the available insulin effectively. In Type 1 diabetes, the pancreas produces no insulin at all. In both scenarios, the result is the same: glucose accumulates in the bloodstream instead of being converted into energy.

Now, you might wonder, "So what?" Well, elevated blood sugar levels can wreak havoc on your body in a variety of ways. Not only can they damage essential organs, but they also raise the risk of severe complications such as kidney failure, heart attack, and strokes. The repercussions can even be as extreme as causing blindness or necessitating limb amputations.

If diabetes is something that has been lurking in your family history, then it's particularly crucial to keep an eye out for symptoms. Far too often, we overlook the warning signs of this condition, despite its potentially severe and life-altering consequences.

It's important to know the subtle changes in your body and seek your medical provider to rule out diabetic conditions. Some changes that you want to be mindful of are constant thirst, frequent urination, fruity-smelling urine, and tiredness. Another sign that can be easily overlooked is the black ring around your toilet, which some mistakenly believe to be a dirty toilet. Indeed, when your blood sugar is high, your body will try to compensate by secreting it out through urine. Overtime, the sugar containing urine can be a great medium for mold to quickly develop and form the black ring around the toilet.

A PERSONAL WAKE-UP CALL

Ten years ago, a moment changed my life and ignited my passion for the topic we're discussing now. My husband came to me complaining of relentless thirst, frequent urination, and unshakeable fatigue. As a nurse, you'd think I'd connect the dots instantly, right? But denial clouded my judgment. It wasn't until a family member mentioned the dreaded word—diabetes—that reality hit me like a ton of bricks. Panicked and worried, I urged my husband to rush to the ER for immediate blood work. My worst fears were confirmed: he was diagnosed with diabetes.

Since that life-altering revelation, I've delved deeply into the subject. Not just because it's personal, but also because I've come to realize how profoundly diabetes can impact our beauty, especially our skin. Stick with me, ladies; we're going on a journey to explore how this condition affects us and, more importantly, how we can fight back.

First of all, I want to relay to you a couple of reminders: If you are a person with diabetes, you must regularly check your blood glucose levels and learn to keep the level under control to prevent complications from developing. Glucose is a natural substance found in food and is converted into energy by the body when it is broken down in the digestive system. Insulin, which is produced by the pancreas, is responsible for allowing the glucose to enter the cells and use it for energy. Unfortunately, if the pancreas does not produce enough insulin, glucose does not get into the cells and accumulates in the blood. This can damage the organs, nerves, and blood vessels.

EARLY SIGNS OF DIABETES: LISTENING TO YOUR BODY

Diabetes often whispers its presence before it shouts, so paying attention to early signs is crucial. Some of the common warning signs include excessive thirst, frequent urination, fatigue, and an inexplicable hunger that doesn't seem to go away. But here's a less-talked-about clue: **dark, velvety patches on the creases of your skin**—such as on the neck, underarms, or groin. This condition, known as acanthosis nigricans, can signal insulin resistance and may be an early indicator of diabetes.

Take a moment to reflect: Have you or someone close to you noticed these symptoms? If so, don't ignore them. Encouraging loved ones to seek medical advice and blood tests promptly can prevent more severe complications. Left unchecked, diabetes can progress to more dangerous conditions like **diabetic ketoacidosis (DKA)**. Symptoms of DKA include dry mouth, flushed face, fruity-smelling breath, headaches, and even nausea or vomiting. From personal experience, I'm grateful I took quick action when my husband showed these symptoms, ensuring he received timely treatment in the emergency room.

For many women, our skin is like a mirror reflecting what's

happening inside our bodies. It tells a story, sometimes whispering signs we might otherwise miss.

Beyond the internal challenges of managing blood sugar levels, diabetes can create noticeable changes in the skin that deserve attention. These changes aren't just cosmetic; they can provide important clues about your health and how well your diabetes is being managed.

Let's dive deeper into the relationship between diabetes and skin health, uncovering what your body may be trying to tell you and how to care for yourself inside and out.

DIABETES AND THE SKIN

The skin is your body's largest organ, and it plays a vital role in how you experience the world—through touch, temperature, and pressure. However, diabetes can interfere with these essential functions, particularly in the feet and ankles. It's not just about how your skin feels, but also how it heals and protects you.

With diabetes, nerve damage and poor blood flow often go hand in hand. You may find yourself losing sensation in your feet. For instance, stepping on a sharp object might go unnoticed, or a small cut or blister might not cause pain or catch your attention. Tight shoes or high heels can create blisters, but without the usual discomfort to alert you, these small issues can spiral into serious infections if left untreated.

Pro Tip: Resist the urge to pop blisters—no matter how tempting it may be! I know, it's hard, but your skin will thank you.

My best advice? Make it a habit to check your skin regularly. Start at your feet—between your toes, around your heels, and up your ankles—then work your way up to your shins and calves. Keep an eye out for anything unusual, like cuts, redness, or swelling. If you spot something, don't wait—bring it to your doctor's attention immediately.

But that's not all. Diabetes doesn't just impact your feet—it can cause a variety of skin conditions, some of which may seem harmless at first glance. While certain issues might clear up on their own, others require prompt medical care. Left untreated, these conditions can escalate into more serious problems.

Remember, poorly controlled blood sugar takes a toll on the small blood vessels in your skin, affecting circulation and its ability to heal. On top of that, a weakened immune system makes even minor cuts or lesions a bigger concern. Your skin is sending you signals—don't ignore them! If something doesn't look or feel right, make that call to your doctor.

DRY AND ITCHY SKIN? BLAME YOUR BLOOD SUGAR!

Dry, itchy skin isn't just an inconvenience—it can be a sign of high blood sugar. My husband often complained of his skin feeling dry, needing constant lotion. Turns out, elevated blood sugar leads to Cytokines circulating in the body. Cytokines are inflammatory elements that can cause itching. There is an association between high Cytokine levels and diabetic nerve damage. So watch out for itchiness! It can indicate more internal health problems than you might think. Diabetes also draws moisture from your skin through frequent urination. Moisturizers specially formulated for diabetics can help, but avoiding hot showers and keeping blood sugar in check is key!

ACANTHOSIS NIGRICANS (AKA THOSE MYSTERIOUS DARK PATCHES)

I know, "Acanthosis Nigricans" sounds like something you'd need a dictionary to understand, but it's actually a common skin condition for people with Type 2 diabetes. When you think "Type 2," think "insulin resistance." Normally, insulin is like a friendly delivery service, making sure sugar gets to your cells for energy. But in diabetics, the deliveries get delayed or do not happen, and sugar just lingers in the bloodstream. At the same time, the insulin level in the blood spikes. Excess insulin triggers skin cells to multiply rapidly. These new cells contain more melanin, resulting in patches of skin that appear darker than the surrounding area. My husband's neck? Yep, sporting one of those patches! Of course, he couldn't see it, so I had to snap a photo to prove it.

If you spot these darker areas, don't waste time on brightening creams. That's your body giving you a heads-up, not a beauty crisis. See a doctor, rule out diabetes, and take action. Remember, it's your health that really counts!

BACTERIAL SKIN INFECTIONS

Let's face it—bacteria is everywhere, and bacterial infections are sneakier than you might think. Unfortunately for diabetics, they tend to be more susceptible to these pesky invaders. Why? Because bacteria *love* sugar, and high blood sugar levels create the perfect all-you-can-eat buffet for them. The most common culprit? Staphylococcus, the bacteria responsible for charming conditions like boils, eyelid styes, lesions, and cellulitis. Not exactly what you'd call a glamorous look, right? And while antibiotics are the go-to treatment, the best medicine is prevention.

The key to avoiding these unwanted guests? Keeping your blood sugar in check! Nobody wants a swollen eyelid or a boil popping up right before a night out with friends. As women, this kind of skin issue can hit us hard. Let's be honest: you'd rather cancel dinner plans than show up with a stye as your plus-one!

Be vigilant with your skin. If you notice warmth, swelling, or tenderness, don't brush it off. Go see a doctor, because with diabetes, even the smallest infection can spiral out of control in no time. Stay one step ahead, and your skin (and social life) will thank you!

FUNGAL INFECTIONS: WHEN SUGAR BECOMES THE PARTY STARTER

Here's a little-known truth: your body is home to a natural ecosystem of microbes, including Candida albicans—a yeast that hangs out in places like your skin, gut, mouth, and, yes, even private areas. Normally, it's just a quiet tenant, but for people with diabetes, it can quickly turn into an unwanted, overzealous party crasher.

Why? High blood sugar doesn't just stay in your bloodstream; it shows up in sweat, saliva, and even urine. For yeast, that's like an all-you-can-eat buffet. This sugar-fueled environment creates the perfect conditions for yeast to overgrow, leading to fungal infections in areas like between your toes, under your armpits, private areas, and even your mouth. Think of it as yeast shouting, "Party time!"—except it's a party you definitely don't want.

Take oral thrush, for example. If you've ever noticed a white, cottage cheese-like coating on your tongue—especially towards the back—and maybe even bad breath to go with it, that's yeast having its moment. Left unchecked, it can spread beyond your mouth, and trust me, you don't want that.

So, what's a proactive woman to do? First, prevention is your best weapon. Keeping your blood sugar levels in check is like shutting down the DJ before the yeast even gets started. Next, rethink your snack habits. Instead of sugary sodas, cakes, or juices loaded with high-fructose corn syrup (yeast's favorite treats), reach for nuts, seeds, fresh fruits, or protein-packed options. A healthier immune system and balanced diet help keep the yeast in its place.

But what if you're already dealing with an infection? Don't wait it out—this is your cue to see a doctor and get the right anti-fungal treatment. Remember, yeast grows fast, and if left unchecked, it can cause more serious issues like bloodstream infections. So, treat it early, treat it right, and treat yourself to the health and confidence you deserve.

Now that we've tackled the fungal front, let's explore other skin conditions diabetics are more prone to—and how you can manage them with grace and care.

DIABETIC DERMOPATHY: WHAT'S UP WITH THOSE MYSTERIOUS SPOTS?

Diabetic dermopathy might sound like a term from a medical textbook, but it's actually quite simple—it refers to small, light brown spots that can appear on your skin, particularly around your shins. These spots can be flat, slightly indented, or oval-shaped, and they vary in size. At first glance, they might look like age spots or marks left behind by a bump or scrape.

I'll never forget the moment I noticed these mysterious brownish spots on my husband's legs. My inner Sherlock Holmes kicked in, trying to piece together the puzzle. "Is this just an early sign of aging?" I thought. But when I learned they were linked to his diabetes, it was an eye-opener. Diabetic dermopathy is often a sign of weakened blood circulation or changes in the small blood vessels due to high blood sugar levels.

The good news? These spots are usually harmless. They don't itch, hurt, or cause any direct discomfort. However—and this is important—they can serve as a subtle signal that something more serious might be happening under the surface, like neuropathy (nerve damage) or retinopathy (eye damage). So, while they might seem like no big deal, they're worth mentioning to your doctor.

Think of these spots as your skin's way of sending you a post-card: "Hey, pay attention to what's going on!" It's a gentle reminder to stay on top of your health and blood sugar management. The next time you notice these marks on your-self or a loved one, don't shrug them off—schedule that doctor's visit. It's always better to be proactive and ensure you're catching any potential complications early. After all, your skin is your body's storyteller, and every mark has a tale to tell.

DIABETES AND BLOOD VESSELS: WHEN THE FLOW GETS SLOW

Diabetes doesn't just mess with your blood sugar—it slows down your blood flow like a clogged drainpipe. Have you heard of *atherosclerosis*? It's when excess sugar causes inflammation, and your artery walls thicken. Imagine trying to get water through a garden hose that's packed with sludge. Not great, right? That's what happens to your blood when it can't flow smoothly.

Think of your blood as the VIP shuttle for your body—delivering oxygen, nutrients, and taking out the trash (waste products). But if it's stuck in traffic, things can get messy fast. Less blood flow means your skin doesn't get the TLC it needs, which leads to dullness and—yep—wrinkles. Worst-case scenario? If blood can't reach your heart or brain, you're looking at serious issues like heart attacks or strokes.

IT'S MORE THAN JUST BLOOD SUGAR

If you think diabetes is just about watching your sugar levels, guess again—it's got its hands in way more than that. High blood sugar can weaken your immune system, slow down healing (even for tiny cuts), and invite infections like unwanted houseguests that won't leave. It's as if your blood vessels are pulling a prank by narrowing down and delivering less oxygen. And it's not just your skin—high glucose can mess with your vision too, leaving you with blurry sight or, in severe cases, blindness.

DIABETES AND PREMATURE AGING: WHY SUGAR IS STEALING YOUR GLOW

Here's a not-so-sweet truth: diabetes can speed up the aging process, and not in the charming "distinguished silver fox" way. High blood sugar levels don't just mess with your health—they also take a toll on your skin. Why? Because when there's too much sugar in your bloodstream, it binds to proteins like collagen and elastin, forming harmful molecules called **Advanced Glycation End Products (AGEs).**

Think of AGEs as sugar-coated wrecking balls. They damage the collagen and elastin fibers that keep your skin firm, smooth, and bouncy. The result? Skin that's dry, dull, and prone to wrinkles. Over time, this glycation process weakens your skin's structure, leading to sagging and fine lines. Basically, instead of rocking a radiant, youthful glow, your skin ends up looking more tired than you feel after a long day.

But here's the good news: you're not powerless. Managing your blood sugar levels can help slow down the glycation process, protecting your skin and keeping those pesky AGEs at bay. Show your skin some love by staying hydrated, eating antioxidant-rich foods, and keeping your skincare routine gentle and nourishing. Products with ingredients like retinol or peptides can help rebuild collagen, while moisturizers with ceramides or hyaluronic acid keep your skin hydrated and supple.

So yes, diabetes can be a challenge, but it doesn't have to define your glow. By managing your blood sugar and giving your skin a little extra TLC, you can stay one step ahead of those AGEs —and age gracefully on your own terms.

While premature aging is one of the many skin changes diabetes can bring, the good news is that there are practical steps you can take to manage and even prevent these issues. Let's dive into some strategies to keep your skin healthy and resilient.

GETTING RELIEF FROM DIABETES-RELATED SKIN PROBLEMS

Managing diabetes-related skin problems requires a proactive and mindful approach. Here's how you can take charge of your skin health while managing your diabetes:

1. **Educate Yourself:** Knowledge is power! Start by speaking with your doctor, reading credible resources, and understanding how diabetes impacts your body, including your skin. The more you know, the better equipped you'll be to prevent and manage skin-related complications.

2. **Check Your Skin Regularly:** Be diligent about inspecting your skin daily, especially those hard-to-reach or less visible areas like your heels, between your toes and fingers, the groin, and armpits. Small issues like cuts, cracks, or irritation can quickly escalate if left unnoticed, so make it a habit to give your skin a quick once-over every day.

3. **Control Your Blood Sugar:** Keeping your blood sugar levels within the normal range is essential for preventing diabetes-related skin issues. Elevated blood sugar not only exacerbates skin problems but also increases the risk of more severe health complications. Work with your healthcare provider to monitor and maintain healthy glucose levels.

4. **Adopt Healthy Lifestyle Habits:** Nourish your body with a balanced diet and make time for regular exercise. These habits not only help manage your weight but also improve circulation and reduce inflammation. If your BMI is creeping into the overweight range, take small steps—like cutting back on salty snacks—to make a difference. Remember, a healthy BMI falls between 18.5 and 24.9, and keeping yours in check is a cornerstone of diabetes management.

5. **Stay Vigilant for Nerve Damage:** Diabetes can lead to nerve damage, making it harder to detect injuries or infections. Pay close attention to your body and check it daily for any signs of trouble, especially in areas that may not feel pain as they should. Early detection can prevent minor issues from becoming major problems.

6. **Treat Wounds and Sores Properly:** If you notice any wounds, sores, or other skin concerns, don't ignore them. Clean and treat them promptly, and if something doesn't seem to be healing or worsens, consult your doctor immediately. Proper wound care can save you from infections and complications.

7. **Hydrate and Moisturize:** Keep your skin hydrated with a good-quality, fragrance-free moisturizer. This helps prevent dryness and cracking, which can become entry points for infections. Drinking plenty of water also supports your skin's health from the inside out.

8. **Protect Your Skin:** Wear protective clothing and sunscreen to shield your skin from harmful UV rays and environmental damage. This is especially important for those with diabetes, as skin can be more sensitive to external factors.

9. **Seek Support:** Managing diabetes isn't something you have to do alone. Join a support group, speak with a dietitian, or work with a diabetes educator to help you navigate the challenges and stay on track with your health goals.

FINAL NOTE

Your skin is your body's first line of defense—it reflects your overall health and needs your care. By staying proactive, controlling your blood sugar, and building a strong foundation of healthy habits, you can minimize the risk of diabetes-related skin problems and live more comfortably. Listen to your body, and don't hesitate to seek professional help when needed. After all, your well-being deserves nothing less than your full attention!

HERBAL HELPERS: BOOSTING YOUR DIABETES DEFENSE WITH NATURAL REMEDIES

You might want to support your diabetes management by taking supplements that contain specific herbs, vitamins, and flavonoids. These natural ingredients work in different ways to help manage blood sugar levels and support overall health. Let's break it down:

Flavonoids: Nature's Powerful Antioxidants

Flavonoids are plant compounds that offer a wide range of health benefits, particularly for diabetics. These compounds help improve blood circulation, support immune function, and reduce inflammation. They also act as antioxidants, neutralizing harmful free radicals that can damage cells. Many herbs used for diabetes management are rich in flavonoids, which can be key in controlling blood sugar and preventing complications.

One specific flavonoid that stands out is Quercetin. Found in many fruits and vegetables, quercetin has shown promise in improving insulin secretion and protecting against damage to blood vessels caused by high blood sugar. It's like a shield for your body, helping to reduce the risks associated with diabetes, including neuropathy and retinopathy. With quercetin on your side, you're not just managing blood sugar—you're proactively protecting your health.

Nature's Secret Allies: Key Herbs for Diabetes Management

Let's talk about nature's pharmacy—a treasure trove of herbs and nutrients that can support you in managing diabetes. These aren't just ingredients; they're like your personal squad of health heroes, each with its unique superpower. Ready to meet the team?

- **Chromium: The Insulin Whisperer.** Think of chromium as insulin's bestie—it helps insulin do its job more effectively. When you have type 2 diabetes, this is a game-changer, helping stabilize those pesky blood sugar spikes that can leave you feeling tired or cranky. Bonus? It might just make those post-meal crashes a thing of the past.
- **Fenugreek Seeds: Small But Mighty.** These little seeds pack a punch. Loaded with fiber, they work like a slow-release system for sugar, helping your body absorb carbs more gradually. Fun fact: research shows that just 1 gram a day can improve insulin sensitivity. Plus, who doesn't love a natural remedy that also helps keep you full longer?
- **Alpha-Lipoic Acid (ALA): The Dual-Action Defender.** ALA doesn't just help manage blood sugar—it's like a shield against nerve damage (hello, diabetic neuropathy). Studies suggest it can even reduce nerve pain. Imagine having a built-in bodyguard for your cells while also keeping your energy levels up.
- **Bilberry Extract: Your Eye's Best Friend.** If you're worried about your vision (and let's face it, screen time doesn't help), bilberry's got your back. It's packed with antioxidants that improve blood flow to the eyes, helping ward off diabetic retinopathy. Think of it as a gentle hug for your eyesight.
- **Bitter Melon: Sweet Benefits, Bitter Taste.** Sure, it's not winning any flavor awards, but bitter melon contains compounds that mimic insulin's effects. It's like nature's way of giving your body a glucose management boost. Pro tip: try it in a stir-fry or as a tea for a more palatable experience.
- **Grape Seed & Pine Bark Extract: The Circulation Champions.** These extracts are your go-to for keeping blood vessels happy and healthy. If you're under 50 and want to safeguard your heart and circulation, they're a must. Think of them as a power

duo that helps prevent complications like high blood pressure.

- **Ginkgo Biloba: The Blood Flow Booster.** Ever feel like your hands and feet are colder than your ex's heart? Ginkgo's here to help! By improving circulation to the extremities and brain, it's perfect for tackling issues like neuropathy and ensuring your nerves stay in tip-top shape.
- **American Ginseng: Stress's Worst Nightmare.** Stress can wreak havoc on blood sugar levels, and American ginseng is like your zen master in a bottle. Studies show it can reduce post-meal blood glucose levels and even improve long-term blood sugar control (HbA1C). Plus, who doesn't want a little extra calm in their life?
- **Garlic & Onions: Everyday Superstars.** They're not just kitchen staples—they're blood sugar and blood pressure regulators, too. Garlic and onions bring flavor and function, helping reduce the risk of heart disease while keeping your meals delicious. It's a win-win!

HOW TO USE THESE NATURAL HELPERS

Incorporating these herbs into your routine doesn't have to feel like homework. Whether it's a pinch of garlic in your dinner, a cup of bitter melon tea, or a daily supplement, the key is consistency. Always check labels and go for quality—your health deserves the best.

How These Herbs Work Together

These herbs and minerals work by targeting multiple aspects of diabetes management. Some help your body use insulin more efficiently (like chromium and fenugreek), while others support your blood vessels and circulation (like ginkgo and grape seed extract). Antioxidants like alpha-lipoic acid and flavonoids such as quercetin provide a protective layer, preventing the damage caused by high blood sugar over time.

So, when you're selecting a supplement, look for one that includes these natural diabetes-fighting ingredients. Together, they form a robust defense team, helping you manage blood sugar, protect your skin, and support overall well-being.

IN SUMMARY: TAKE CHARGE OF YOUR HEALTH AND SKIN

Diabetes doesn't have to control you—your health and beauty are still yours to own!

Let's face it: we've all had our ups and downs with skin issues, whether it was the dreaded teenage acne or the occasional flare-ups that make us feel less than our best. But when diabetes enters the picture, skin changes can feel like yet another hurdle to overcome. The truth is, these changes are often subtle or seem temporary, making them easy to ignore—but this is where we, as women, need to stand up and take notice.

Your skin is your body's largest organ, a living, breathing canvas that reflects your internal health. It's your first line of defense and a messenger, quietly telling you when something's off. Paying close attention to its signals isn't vanity—it's self-care in its most empowering form.

Action Steps: Own Your Wellness Journey

- **Prioritize Self-Care:** Commit to a daily skin-check ritual. From your toes to your scalp, give your body the attention it deserves. Early detection of any changes is your greatest ally.
- **Nurture from Within:** Balance blood sugar levels, stay hydrated, and nourish your body with wholesome foods and targeted supplements. Remember, beauty begins from the inside out.
- **Be Proactive, Not Reactive:** Don't brush off "small" symptoms or temporary-looking changes.

When it comes to diabetes, prevention and early intervention are everything.
- **Seek Support:** Whether it's from your doctor, a nutritionist, or loved ones, lean on your community. Managing diabetes is a team effort, and you don't have to do it alone.
- **Reclaim Your Confidence:** Diabetes might shape how you manage your health, but it doesn't define your beauty. Wear your skin proudly and treat it with the love and care it deserves.

A FINAL NOTE FOR WOMEN

We're more than our diagnoses. We're mothers, daughters, partners, and friends, navigating life's challenges with strength and grace. Let this chapter serve as a reminder that health and beauty aren't mutually exclusive. By taking charge of your diabetes, you're not just improving your skin—you're reclaiming your power, your vibrance, and your confidence.

Ladies, you've got this. Your skin, your health, your story—it's all yours to shine. ✧

CHAPTER 12

THE HEART OF WELLNESS: NURTURING YOUR GUT FOR WHOLE-BODY HEALTH

HEAL YOUR GUT, UNLOCK YOUR GLOW— THE SECRET TO LASTING BEAUTY

WHY GUT HEALTH MATTERS

The idea of "gut health" might seem a bit scientific, but let's think of it as the foundation of feeling good, looking good, and living with vitality. Imagine your gut as the bustling center of a lively city—it has the power to keep everything else in balance when it's running smoothly. And for women, gut health has a profound influence on our entire well-being, from mental clarity to immunity, and even skin and mood!

A little personal story to kick this off: I've had my fair share of "gut issues." During a particularly stressful season in my life, I started noticing a few unsettling changes—my skin was breaking out more than usual, I felt anxious over the smallest things, and my energy levels were wildly unpredictable. At first, I blamed these changes on everything else—work stress, lack of sleep, even the weather! But deep down, I knew something bigger was at play.

That's when I stumbled across the concept of gut health and decided to dig deeper. I began making small changes—adding more fiber to my meals, incorporating fermented foods like yogurt and kimchi, and drinking more water. I even started taking a high-quality probiotic supplement, which felt like giving my gut the VIP treatment it desperately needed.

The results? Nothing short of transformative. My skin cleared up like it had been through a rejuvenation spa, my energy became more consistent, and, surprisingly, my mood improved. It was as if my body was finally thanking me for paying attention to its needs. What I realized is that nurturing your gut doesn't just affect your digestion—it can be the secret to whole-body wellness.

In this chapter, we'll dive into the science of why gut health matters, the signs that your gut might need some TLC, and actionable steps you can take to nurture it. If you've ever felt out of sync with your body, this might just be the chapter that connects the dots for you. Let's explore how taking care of your gut can transform the way you feel and glow, from the inside out!

SECTION 1: THE GUT'S SURPRISING IMPACT ON THE REST OF YOU

Mental Health and Mood: The Surprising Source of Happiness

Did you know that around 90% of your body's serotonin—the so-called "feel-good" hormone—is produced in your gut, not your brain? Most people think serotonin is all about the brain, but the intestines are the real production powerhouse.

So, what exactly is serotonin?

Serotonin is a neurotransmitter, or chemical messenger, that helps regulate a whole range of essential functions like mood, sleep, appetite, and even memory. Often dubbed the "happy hormone," it's like the conductor of your emotional symphony, creating feelings of calm, positivity, and well-being.

Why Serotonin is Produced in the Gut

Here's something surprising: your gut doesn't just digest food—it plays a starring role in your mood. Around 90% of the body's serotonin, often called the "feel-good" hormone, is produced in your gut, not your brain. That's because your gut houses its own "mini-brain," known as the enteric nervous system, which constantly chats with your brain via the gut-brain axis—a two-way communication highway.

When your gut microbiome—the community of good bacteria in your intestines—is balanced, serotonin production runs like a well-oiled machine, helping boost mood, improve mental clarity, and promote emotional stability. On the flip side, an imbalanced gut can disrupt serotonin levels, potentially leading to mood swings, anxiety, or depression. Think of your gut as the cheerleader for your happiness—keeping it healthy keeps your spirits high.

Immunity: Your Gut's Role as a Bodyguard

Your gut isn't just about digestion—it's your immune system's headquarters, housing about 70% of the body's immune cells. Why? Because the gut is the body's frontline defense, constantly exposed to potential threats from the food and water we consume. To protect us, immune cells line the gut wall, ready to neutralize harmful bacteria, viruses, and toxins.

When your gut microbiome is balanced, it bolsters your immune response, reducing your chances of catching illnesses like the common cold. But an unbalanced gut can weaken these defenses, leaving you more vulnerable to infections and chronic inflammation. Keeping your gut healthy isn't just about digestion—it's about strengthening your body's natural armor.

Hormonal Harmony: Gut Health as the Silent Regulator

Hormones control everything from mood and metabolism to skin and energy. While we often focus on glands like the thyroid or adrenal glands, your gut also plays a major role in hormone regulation.

- **Leptin and hunger cues:** A healthy gut helps regulate leptin, the hormone that tells you when you're full. When your gut is balanced, leptin levels stay steady, reducing cravings and helping you feel satisfied after meals. But an unbalanced gut can disrupt leptin, leading to overeating and a desire for sugary or processed foods.
- **Weight management:** Your gut microbiome affects how efficiently your body metabolizes food and stores energy. A balanced gut supports healthy digestion and weight, while an imbalanced gut might encourage weight gain by promoting cravings for calorie-dense, nutrient-poor foods.
- **Skin health:** Hormonal imbalances often show up on your skin in the form of acne, redness, or other irritations. The gut-skin axis is real—when your gut is healthy, your hormones are more stable, leading to clearer, more radiant skin.

Digestive Wellness: The Gut as Your Internal Guide

Your gut is like a built-in nutrition coach. When balanced, it sends clear signals to your brain about what your body needs, making you crave wholesome, nourishing foods. An unbalanced gut, however, can hijack these signals, pushing you toward sugary or fatty snacks and leaving you hungry soon after.

Imagine this: after a balanced meal, you feel full, energized, and satisfied. Contrast that with a processed, high-sugar meal that leaves you reaching for a snack an hour later. That's your gut influencing your cravings and satiety. By keeping your gut in balance, you're setting yourself up for better digestion, healthier choices, and sustained energy.

Skin Health: The Gut's Radiant Reflection

Your gut isn't just a partner in digestion—it's a key player in your skincare routine. The gut-skin axis links the health of your gut microbiome to inflammation levels in your body, which directly affect your skin's appearance. When your gut is balanced, inflammation is reduced, leading to fewer breakouts and a brighter complexion. But when your gut is off-balance, inflammation rises, potentially causing acne, redness, or conditions like eczema.

Studies have found that people with clear skin tend to have a healthier gut microbiome compared to those with chronic skin issues. Think of gut health as your "inner glow-up." By nourishing your gut, you're not just promoting better digestion—you're enhancing your natural beauty from the inside out.

SECTION 2: GUT HEALTH AND REGULARITY – WHY A SMOOTH ROUTINE MATTERS

Let's talk about something not-so-glamorous but oh-so-important: regularity. A healthy gut isn't just about what you eat or your mood—it's also about how well everything "moves" along in your digestive system. Constipation can disrupt that flow, affecting not only your comfort but also the very health of your gut environment.

Constipation and Toxin Buildup: The Hidden Consequence

Did you know that constipation can lead to toxin buildup in the gut? When things slow down, waste sits in the colon longer than it should. Not only is this uncomfortable, but it also allows certain toxins to be reabsorbed into the body, which can cause inflammation and strain gut health. Picture it as a traffic jam that keeps waste piling up, creating a cascade of not-so-pleasant effects on your overall well-being.

Gut Microbiome Imbalance: The Root of Bloating and Discomfort

Constipation doesn't just stop things up; it also disrupts the delicate balance of good and bad bacteria in your gut. Waste lingering in your intestines creates the perfect environment for harmful bacteria to multiply, crowding out the friendly bacteria that play essential roles in digestion, immunity, and overall health.

Here's the science: as bad bacteria feed on undigested food—especially carbohydrates—they produce gas as a byproduct. This gas builds up, causing bloating, discomfort, and that all-too-familiar "puffy" feeling. And while bad bacteria aren't necessarily causing infections during constipation, they can trigger inflammation by releasing toxins that irritate the gut lining.

What's more, this imbalance doesn't just affect your digestive system—it impacts your mood and energy. Thanks to the gut-brain axis, an unhappy gut can send stress signals to your brain, leaving you feeling cranky, sluggish, or just "off." Essentially, when your gut struggles, so do you.

Mood, Immune Health, and Regularity: It's All Connected

Your gut has a powerful connection to your brain (remember that serotonin we talked about?) and to your immune system. When constipation throws off the gut's balance, it doesn't just affect digestion—it can spark an inflammatory response in your body, further impacting how you feel emotionally and physically.

Regularity ensures that waste is moving along efficiently, preventing toxin buildup and keeping your microbiome in harmony. A happy, well-functioning gut means stronger immunity, more stable moods, and an overall sense of balance in your body.

SECTION 3: YOUR ACTION PLAN FOR A HAPPY, HEALTHY GUT

Supporting gut health doesn't have to be complicated or boring —it's about making small, thoughtful choices every day that help your digestive system thrive. From balancing your microbiome to preventing constipation, here's your step-by-step guide to gut bliss:

1. Stick to a Consistent Eating Schedule

Your gut thrives on routine, much like a well-tuned orchestra. Eating meals at the same time every day helps regulate your digestive processes, aligning them with your body's natural circadian rhythms. Think of it as setting your gut's internal clock—breakfast at 8 a.m., lunch at 12 p.m., and dinner at 6 p.m. This predictability allows your digestive system to prepare for meals, ensuring smoother digestion, reducing bloating, and keeping hunger hormones like ghrelin and leptin in check. When meals are eaten at erratic times, it's like the orchestra is out of sync, creating chaos in your gut. A consistent eating schedule is like giving your gut a daily high-five, setting the stage for better digestion, balanced energy, and overall gut harmony.

2. Embrace the Prebiotics and Probiotics Combo

Your gut loves balance, and prebiotics and probiotics are the dream team:

Probiotics: These live bacteria are like your gut's cheerleaders. Load up on yogurt, kefir, kimchi, and sauerkraut to introduce beneficial bacteria that aid digestion.

Prebiotics: These are the fibers that feed your good bacteria, keeping them thriving. Foods like garlic, onions, bananas, and asparagus are easy (and delicious) ways to fuel your microbiome. Bonus points for an apple a day—it really does keep the doctor away!

3. Fuel Up with Fiber

Fiber is your gut's best friend when it comes to regularity. Foods like oats, chia seeds, leafy greens, and whole grains not only keep things moving but also help nourish your gut bacteria. Remember: add fiber gradually and pair it with plenty of water —fiber without hydration is like a car without gas!

4. Hydrate Like It's Your Job

Water is the unsung hero of digestion. It helps soften stool, prevent constipation, and keep your digestive system running smoothly. A simple rule: If you're thirsty, your gut is already feeling parched. Keep a water bottle handy and sip consistently throughout the day.

5. Say Yes to Fermented Foods

Fermented foods like kombucha, miso, pickles, and tempeh bring diversity to your gut microbiome. Even a small serving— a spoonful of sauerkraut or a cup of kombucha—can make a big difference. Your gut bacteria will thank you with better digestion and a stronger immune system.

6. Mindful Eating: Chew and Savor

Slow down! Eating too quickly can overwhelm your gut and lead to bloating or discomfort. Take time to chew thoroughly and enjoy your meal—it gives your digestive system a head start and allows your brain to catch up with fullness signals. Bonus: it's also a great way to savor your favorite flavors.

7. Incorporate Natural Laxative Foods

Feeling backed up? Nature's got your back. Prunes, pears, and kiwi are gentle, effective options for promoting regularity without resorting to harsh solutions. Plus, they're sweet and delicious—a win-win for your gut and your taste buds.

8. Move Your Body, Move Your Gut

Exercise isn't just about looking good—it's about keeping your digestive system on track. Even a 20-minute brisk walk can help stimulate your gut and encourage regular bowel movements. Yoga and stretching can also ease bloating and discomfort.

9. Replenish After Antibiotics

Antibiotics are sometimes necessary, but they can wreak havoc on your gut microbiome. Replenish your good bacteria with probiotic-rich foods or a high-quality probiotic supplement to restore balance and support recovery.

10. Manage Stress and Prioritize Sleep

Stress and poor sleep can throw your gut into chaos. Practices like meditation, journaling, or deep breathing exercises can help calm your mind—and your gut. Sleep is also a key player; aim for 7-9 hours of quality rest to give your digestive system the downtime it needs to repair and regenerate.

11. Limit Gut Disruptors

Too much alcohol or caffeine can irritate your gut and disrupt its balance. Enjoy these in moderation, and always pair them with plenty of water and nutrient-rich foods to offset potential harm.

12. Natural Oils for Gentle Relief

If constipation becomes a persistent issue, consider incorporating natural oils like olive oil, coconut oil, or flaxseed oil. Just a tablespoon in the morning can act as a gentle lubricant for your digestive system, helping to get things moving.

FINAL THOUGHT: TREAT YOUR GUT LIKE YOUR BEST FRIEND

Your gut works hard for you every day—so why not return the favor? By maintaining a consistent eating schedule, nourishing it with the right foods, staying active, and managing stress, you can create a happy, healthy environment for your gut to thrive. And when your gut is happy, trust me, the rest of your body will follow suit!

CONCLUSION: A GUT FEELING YOU CAN TRUST—FROM THE INSIDE OUT

Taking care of your gut isn't just about digestion—it's the foundation of your health, vitality, and confidence as a woman. It's the starting point for mental clarity, balanced moods, glowing skin, strong immunity, and even hormonal harmony. When your gut is in balance, your entire body thrives.

Imagine waking up with steady energy, a radiant complexion, and a calm, clear mind—knowing that the small, intentional habits you've adopted are shaping a stronger, healthier you. By sticking to a routine, choosing gut-friendly foods, hydrating, and practicing mindfulness, you're not just improving digestion; you're building a life in which you feel vibrant, resilient, and unstoppable.

This is your moment to reclaim your health, one mindful step at a time. Treat your gut like the powerful ally it is. With every meal, every sip of water, and every moment of care, you're creating a ripple effect of wellness that starts from within and radiates outward. You've got this—because when your gut is happy, you are unstoppable.

CHAPTER 13
WEIGHT LOSS UNLOCKED
THE JOURNEY TO HEALTH, CONFIDENCE, AND LASTING CHANGE

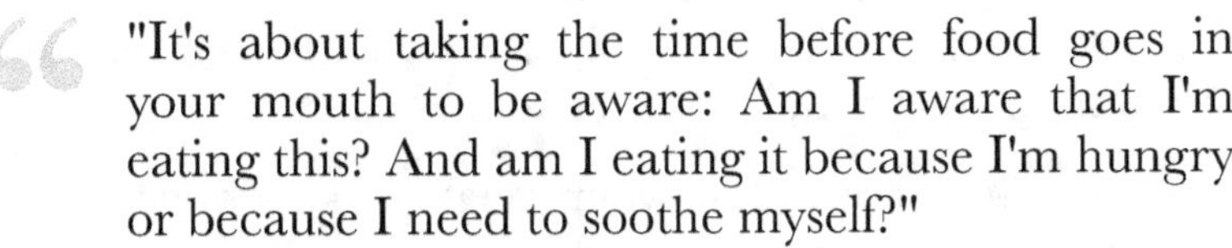

"It's about taking the time before food goes in your mouth to be aware: Am I aware that I'm eating this? And am I eating it because I'm hungry or because I need to soothe myself?"

— Valerie Bertinelli

In today's world, where "self-love" and body positivity are celebrated, the topic of weight can feel like a sensitive subject to tackle. But let's be honest: while self-acceptance is empowering, there's an undeniable connection between our weight and our overall health. As a nurse, I've seen how carrying extra pounds can quietly lead to serious health challenges—issues that often creep up unnoticed until they're unavoidable.

Did you know that more than a third of adults in the United States are classified as obese, according to the CDC? Beyond the numbers, though, there's a deeper question: how is your weight affecting the way you feel, the way you live, and even the way you see yourself? Weight is more than just a number on the scale—it's intertwined with our physical health, emotional well-being, and even our outward appearance.

In this chapter, we'll explore the realities of weight—not with judgment or pressure, but with curiosity, care, and practical steps to find balance. Let's discover how shedding the physical and emotional weight can lead to a lighter, more vibrant version of you.

DECODING BMI: MORE THAN JUST A NUMBER

Alright, let's talk numbers—specifically, the one that sparks either relief or mild panic for many of us: BMI, or Body Mass Index. You've probably heard of it, but what is it really? Think of BMI as the mathematical lovechild of your height and weight. Healthcare professionals use it to give a rough estimate of whether you fall into the "healthy weight," "overweight," or "obese" category. It's like a friendly, somewhat flawed tool that tries to sum up your body in one neat little number.

The calculation is simple: take your weight in kilograms, divide it by your height in meters squared, and voilà—your BMI. But before you grab a calculator, let's add a dose of reality: while useful, BMI is far from perfect.

Here's why. Imagine you're an athlete with lean muscle and barely any body fat, or perhaps you've been killing it at strength training. Despite being in incredible shape, your BMI might place you in the "overweight" or even "obese" range. Why? Because BMI doesn't differentiate between fat and muscle—it only sees the total weight. So yes, you could be rocking a sculpted physique, but BMI might still treat you like you've spent one too many evenings indulging in dessert.

And then there's bone density. If you're naturally solidly built, BMI won't give you extra credit for that, either. It lumps everyone into the same categories, ignoring whether your "extra" weight comes from muscle, bone, or something else entirely.

In short, BMI is like that well-meaning friend who oversimplifies everything. It offers a general idea of where you stand but doesn't tell the full story. Your health is so much more than a single number—it's a reflection of your habits, diet, exercise routine, and overall lifestyle. So, if your BMI isn't where you want it to be, don't panic. Instead, take a breath and remember: health is a much bigger picture than one quirky formula can capture.

THE WEIGHT OF OBESITY: A STRAIN ON PHYSICAL HEALTH

Carrying extra weight places a significant strain on our bodies in countless ways, affecting everything from joint health to organ function. Working as a surgery case manager in an orthopedic clinic, I've seen firsthand how the majority of patients undergoing knee or hip replacements are overweight. Joint pain is a common complaint among individuals carrying excess weight because joints are forced to bear more stress than they were designed to handle. Over time, this constant strain can lead to arthritis or worsen existing conditions. Here's the good news: losing even a small amount of weight can reduce joint pain, improve mobility, and potentially save you from needing invasive surgeries like knee replacements.

Obesity doesn't just impact your joints; it also significantly increases your risk of developing life-threatening conditions such as heart disease, stroke, high blood pressure, and diabetes. In fact, obesity-related diseases rank among the leading causes of preventable death in the United States.

Now let's talk about the toll extra weight takes on your organs. Imagine carrying a heavy backpack everywhere—it's exhausting, right? That's what your body experiences when it's dealing with excess fat, especially around the chest, neck, and abdomen. For your lungs, this additional weight restricts their ability to expand fully, making it harder to breathe deeply and worsening conditions like asthma or sleep apnea. Similarly, your kidneys face extra pressure and are forced to work overtime. Over time, this stress can lead to decreased kidney function and serious complications.

Knowing these impacts, it's time to become more self-aware. Noticed a few extra pounds creeping on? That's your cue to take intentional action. By shedding even a small amount of weight, you can alleviate the strain on your body, improve your quality of life, and invest in your future health. Remember, every step toward a healthier you is a step worth taking.

OBESITY AND SKIN HEALTH: THE CONNECTION YOU DIDN'T EXPECT

There's a Vietnamese saying that goes something like this: "First comes your figure, then comes your skin." For many women, the ideal vision of beauty is a slim, curvy body paired with glowing, flawless skin. While that may sound dreamy, what often gets overlooked is the strong connection between weight and skin health. Let's unpack why this happens and what you can do about it.

Obesity doesn't just affect your physical health—it can have a significant impact on your skin as well. Carrying extra weight often leads to chronic inflammation, which can show up as acne, psoriasis, or other skin issues. Fat tissue, especially in areas with skin folds, creates friction, leading to irritation, rashes, or even fungal infections. If you've ever dealt with redness or discomfort in these areas, you know how frustrating it can be.

Hormonal imbalances triggered by being overweight can also play havoc on your skin. Higher levels of certain hormones may cause oily skin and clogged pores, resulting in more frequent breakouts. And then there's the reality of stretch marks. Excess weight stretches the skin to its limits, leading to sagging and those silvery lines that can feel like they're there to stay.

But here's the good news: your skin is resilient. While obesity can negatively impact your skin's health, taking steps toward a healthier weight can help improve its appearance and vitality. Reducing inflammation through proper diet, hydration, and weight management can lead to clearer, healthier-looking skin. Even small lifestyle changes can make a noticeable difference over time.

And let's not overlook the mental health aspect. When we don't feel confident in our bodies, it's easy to let self-doubt creep in, affecting how we see ourselves and interact with others. Low self-esteem and a negative self-image can become heavy burdens, but here's the truth: your worth isn't defined by a number on the scale. No matter your size, you are deserving of love and respect—starting with self-love.

Obesity may pose challenges, but it's something you can address with patience and care. Remember, every step you take toward improving your well-being is a step toward a healthier, more vibrant you. It's not just about looking good; it's about feeling good inside and out. Your journey to better health is also a journey to healthier, glowing skin.

THE HIDDEN LINK BETWEEN OBESITY AND DEPRESSION: BREAKING FREE FROM THE CYCLE

Carrying extra weight doesn't just strain your body—it weighs heavily on your heart and mind, too. Many of us know that sinking feeling when our favorite jeans don't fit or when we avoid the mirror altogether. It's more than just a physical struggle; it's deeply emotional, cutting into our confidence and self-worth. And in a world dominated by beauty filters and picture-perfect Instagram posts, the pressure to look flawless can feel overwhelming. This relentless comparison often feeds feelings of inadequacy, creating a cycle of dissatisfaction that can lead to—or worsen—depression.

The connection between obesity and depression runs deeper than we might realize. Physically, carrying excess weight is draining. It zaps your energy, leaving you too exhausted to enjoy activities that once brought you joy—whether it's playing with your kids, going out with friends, or even savoring a quiet walk in nature. Over time, this fatigue and frustration can turn even simple tasks into monumental challenges, further chipping away at your sense of vitality.

Emotionally, the toll is profound. Weight struggles often come with body image issues and negative self-talk: "I'm not enough" or "I don't deserve to feel good." These voices grow louder, amplifying sadness, loneliness, and a sense of worthlessness. It's not just about the weight itself; it's about how it makes you feel in your own skin. And that feeling can be a heavy burden to carry.

The social aspect compounds the issue. Studies show that people struggling with obesity are less likely to engage in social activities and are more likely to face stigma, bullying, or discrimination. This isolation creates a vicious cycle—feeling disconnected from others worsens mental health, and poor mental health can make it even harder to take steps toward physical wellness.

But here's the truth: your worth isn't tied to a number on the scale. Breaking free from this cycle starts with treating yourself with kindness and compassion. It's about shifting the focus from "what's wrong with me" to "what can I do to feel better?" Small, intentional steps—like seeking support, finding joy in movement, or nourishing your body with love—can make all the difference.

This journey isn't just about shedding pounds; it's about reclaiming your confidence, reconnecting with your joy, and remembering that you are so much more than your reflection in the mirror. Healing takes time, but every step you take toward valuing yourself is a step toward brighter days—inside and out.

REAL-LIFE STORIES: CASE STUDIES IN WEIGHT LOSS

Weight loss is a deeply personal journey, and no two people experience it the same way. By looking at the struggles and triumphs of women who've faced their own weight challenges, we can uncover valuable lessons. These stories remind us that whether it's hormonal imbalances, emotional eating, or the body's natural signals pushing back, the key to success lies in understanding your body and making sustainable, mindful changes.

CASE STUDY 1: SARAH'S STRUGGLE WITH YO-YO DIETING

Sarah, a busy mom of two, had tried every diet under the sun —keto, fasting, low-carb. Each time she started a new plan, the results were immediate. She would lose 5, 10, even 15 pounds in the first month. But after a few months, the progress would unravel. Exhaustion set in, sweet cravings hit hard, and emotionally, she felt drained. Soon enough, the weight crept back, and she found herself in a cycle of binge eating. The stricter her diet, the louder her cravings became, leaving her right back where she started—sometimes even heavier.

Sarah's story is a reflection of a common struggle: yo-yo dieting. Restrictive diets can initially seem like magic because they drastically cut calories or eliminate entire food groups, shocking the system into quick weight loss. But over time, Sarah's body rebelled. Her energy plummeted, hunger signals became impossible to ignore, and cravings turned into uncontrollable binges. This was her body's way of crying out for balance, as extreme diets often deprive it of essential nutrients.

After years of frustration, Sarah made a life-changing decision to shift her mindset. Instead of chasing quick fixes, she began practicing intuitive eating, a method that prioritizes listening to her body's natural hunger and fullness cues. She stopped labeling foods as "good" or "bad" and instead focused on eating in moderation and choosing nutrient-dense meals that made her feel good. By prioritizing balance over restriction, Sarah not only lost weight steadily but also found peace with food and gained control over her emotional relationship with eating.

Key Takeaway from Sarah's Journey:

Your body isn't your enemy; it's trying to protect you. Restrictive diets may deliver short-term results, but they often come at the cost of long-term sustainability. The real win is finding an approach that works with your body, not against it. Intuitive eating, combined with mindfulness, can be a game-changer for both physical health and emotional well-being.

CASE STUDY 2: MARIA'S JOURNEY WITH WEIGHT AND HORMONAL BALANCE

Maria, a 38-year-old working mother, began noticing her weight steadily creeping up after the birth of her second child. She tried cutting calories and experimenting with different workout routines, but no matter what she did, the scale refused to budge. Her frustration grew as the extra pounds left her feeling sluggish and disconnected from her usual vibrant self. To make matters worse, Maria started experiencing irregular periods, which further hinted that something was amiss.

After consulting her doctor, Maria learned that her struggles were tied to hormonal imbalances, specifically elevated levels of cortisol—commonly known as the stress hormone. For women, cortisol can be a sneaky culprit behind stubborn weight gain, particularly around the belly area. When the body is under constant stress, cortisol rises, signaling the body to store fat for "emergencies." Maria's high-pressure job, combined with the endless demands of raising two young children, had created the perfect storm for chronic stress and disrupted hormones.

Maria's breakthrough came when she shifted her focus to stress management rather than extreme dieting or overexercising. She started practicing yoga and mindfulness meditation, making it a non-negotiable part of her daily routine. These calming practices helped reduce her cortisol levels, allowing her body to finally relax and stop clinging to stored fat.

She also revamped her diet, prioritizing whole, nutrient-dense foods that supported her hormonal health. Her meals included lean proteins, healthy fats like avocado and olive oil, and plenty of fiber-rich vegetables and whole grains. Maria was careful to avoid processed foods and sugar, which can exacerbate hormonal imbalances.

Within a few months, Maria began to see and feel a transformation. Her energy levels improved, her mood stabilized, and her weight gradually started to come off—especially in the areas where cortisol had previously taken a toll. More importantly, she felt empowered, realizing that understanding her hormones and stress triggers was key to unlocking her health and weight goals.

Key Takeaway from Maria's Journey:

Stress and hormones play a huge role in weight management, especially for women juggling busy lives. Elevated cortisol levels can make weight loss feel impossible, but focusing on stress-reducing practices and eating for hormonal health can create a dramatic shift. Maria's story reminds us that weight loss isn't just about calories in and calories out—it's about nurturing your body and mind to achieve balance.

CASE STUDY 3: ASHLEY'S JOURNEY WITH EMOTIONAL EATING

For Ashley, a 24-year-old student, food wasn't just nourishment—it became her emotional crutch. Whenever she felt stressed, overwhelmed, or sad, she turned to her favorite comfort foods for relief, even when she wasn't physically hungry. Over time, this habit turned into emotional eating, where food became a way to soothe negative emotions rather than to fuel her body. As a result, Ashley began gaining weight, and her body's natural homeostatic signals—those built-in cues that tell us when we're truly hungry or full—were thrown off balance.

The cycle became a vicious one: the more she ate to cope, the more guilt and frustration she felt, which only led to more emotional eating. It wasn't just about the weight gain; it was the sense of losing control over her health and her relationship with food that weighed on her the most.

Ashley's turning point came when she decided to take a step back and address the root cause of her eating habits—her emotions. She began practicing mindful eating, a technique that encouraged her to slow down, check in with her feelings, and ask herself key questions before eating, such as:

Am I truly hungry, or am I just trying to numb my emotions?

Will this food nourish my body, or am I seeking temporary comfort?

By learning to distinguish between emotional hunger and physical hunger, Ashley started breaking the cycle. She also sought out alternative ways to process her emotions, like journaling, taking a walk, or talking to a friend, instead of reaching for food. Over time, she noticed that her cravings for comfort foods diminished, her weight stabilized, and she felt more in control of her health and emotions.

Key Takeaway from Ashley's Journey:

Emotional eating can be a tough habit to break, but it's not impossible. The first step is recognizing when you're eating to satisfy emotional needs rather than physical hunger. By practicing mindful eating and finding non-food ways to cope with stress and emotions, you can reclaim control over your relationship with food. Ashley's story is a powerful reminder that understanding your emotional triggers and taking small, intentional steps can lead to lasting change—not just for your weight, but for your overall well-being.

CASE STUDY 4: LISA'S TRANSFORMATION THROUGH GUT HEALTH

For Lisa, weight loss felt like a never-ending uphill battle. No matter how hard she pushed herself at the gym or how many diets she tried, the scale barely budged. Beyond the weight, she also dealt with constant bloating, irregular digestion, and low energy—issues that left her feeling defeated and disconnected from her body.

After some deep diving into health research, Lisa stumbled upon a revelation: her gut health might be the missing puzzle piece. The more she learned, the clearer it became—an imbalanced gut microbiome could be slowing her metabolism and making weight loss feel impossible.

Lisa decided to take action. She started introducing probiotic-rich foods into her daily routine, like yogurt, sauerkraut, and kombucha, to replenish the "good" bacteria in her gut. She paired this with prebiotic foods such as oats, garlic, and bananas to nourish those healthy bacteria. Slowly but surely, she noticed a shift—her digestion became smoother, the bloating eased, and her energy levels soared.

With her gut back in balance, her metabolism began functioning more efficiently. Without resorting to extreme measures, Lisa started shedding pounds and, for the first time in years, felt truly in sync with her body. She found herself enjoying the process of nourishing her gut and realized that weight loss wasn't just about the calories in or out; it was about creating harmony within her body.

Key Takeaway from Lisa's Journey:

Sometimes, weight struggles aren't about lack of effort but about deeper, hidden factors like gut health. Lisa's story underscores how critical a balanced microbiome is for efficient metabolism and overall wellness. By focusing on healing her gut, Lisa unlocked her body's natural ability to lose weight and feel energized. Her transformation is a powerful reminder that nurturing your gut isn't just about better digestion—it's about unlocking a healthier, happier version of yourself.

CASE STUDY 5: EMILY'S STRUGGLE WITH HOMEOSTASIS AND WEIGHT LOSS

Emily, a 32-year-old marketing executive, was no stranger to the grind. She counted calories meticulously, stuck to a rigid workout routine, and even experimented with the latest diet trends. Yet, despite her disciplined approach, her weight wouldn't budge. Frustrated and confused, Emily began to feel like her body was working against her, leaving her discouraged and drained.

After consulting with her doctor, Emily learned that her body had hit a homeostasis wall—a state where the body strives to maintain balance and resist change. When we drastically cut calories or overwork ourselves, the body perceives it as a threat and switches into "survival mode." For Emily, this meant her metabolism slowed down to conserve energy, while her hunger hormones, like ghrelin, surged, leaving her constantly hungry. It was a vicious cycle of deprivation and resistance.

The turning point came when Emily stopped fighting her body and started working with it. Instead of focusing on restrictive measures, she adopted small, sustainable habits that supported her body's natural rhythms. She incorporated more strength training into her workouts, which helped build lean muscle and boosted her resting metabolism. Emily also shifted her meals to include more protein, fiber, and healthy fats, ensuring her body felt fueled and satisfied without triggering those survival-mode signals.

As she embraced these changes, Emily noticed her body gradually adapting. Her metabolism started to stabilize, her energy levels improved, and she began to lose weight steadily—not rapidly, but consistently. Most importantly, Emily felt stronger, healthier, and more in tune with her body than ever before.

Key Takeaway from Emily's Journey:

Weight loss isn't about waging war on your body; it's about building trust and balance. Emily's story highlights the importance of understanding homeostasis and the body's natural responses to stress and deprivation. By focusing on sustainable habits, nourishing her body, and respecting its cues, Emily achieved results that felt natural and lasting. Her journey is a reminder that patience, self-care, and a balanced approach are the real keys to long-term success.

WHAT WE CAN LEARN FROM THESE STORIES

These real-life stories illustrate that while every weight loss journey is personal and unique, there are universal lessons that can guide us toward lasting success. Whether it's breaking free from yo-yo dieting like Sarah, tackling hormonal imbalances like Maria, addressing emotional eating like Ashley, supporting gut health like Lisa, or working with your body's natural signals like Emily, each story reveals powerful insights into the complex relationship between our bodies and weight.

Key Takeaways from Each Journey:

- **Sarah's lesson:** Your body isn't the enemy—listen to it. Intuitive eating and avoiding restrictive diets can help you create a healthier, more balanced relationship with food.
- **Maria's lesson:** Stress and hormones are silent players in weight gain. Managing them through relaxation, balanced nutrition, and self-care is key to long-term success.
- **Ashley's lesson:** Food shouldn't be a coping mechanism. Addressing emotional triggers and practicing mindful eating can break the cycle of emotional eating.

- **Lisa's lesson:** Your gut is your weight-loss ally. Supporting your microbiome with probiotics, prebiotics, and balanced meals can rev up your metabolism and improve digestion.
- **Emily's lesson:** Sustainable weight loss isn't about deprivation. Understand and respect your body's homeostasis by making gradual, sustainable changes that work with—not against—your natural rhythms.

How These Lessons Apply to You

These stories remind us that weight loss is not just about the number on the scale—it's about building a healthier, happier life that aligns with your body's unique needs. Each journey reflects the importance of self-awareness, patience, and the power of small, intentional changes. By understanding your body and focusing on sustainable habits, you can overcome obstacles and achieve lasting results.

MOVING FORWARD: BUILDING YOUR OWN SUCCESS STORY

As we dive deeper into this chapter, we'll explore practical strategies inspired by these stories. From intuitive eating to stress management, from gut health tips to understanding homeostasis, you'll learn actionable steps to build your own path to success. Remember: your journey is yours alone, but the lessons from others can serve as a guide. Together, these insights empower us to approach weight loss with confidence, compassion, and the determination to thrive—not just survive.

With the right mindset, a little patience, and the willingness to adapt, you can turn your story into one of transformation, health, and happiness.

WHAT WENT WRONG WITH OUR INNATE GUIDANCE SYSTEM?

Human bodies are beautifully wired with natural signals—homeostatic signals—designed to maintain balance. These signals, powered by hormones like ghrelin (the hunger hormone) and leptin (the satiety hormone), tell us when to eat and when to stop. For early humans, this system worked seamlessly to ensure survival during cycles of feast and famine. When food was scarce, ghrelin would rise, encouraging eating; when full, leptin would kick in, signaling the brain to stop.

Fast forward to today, where food is everywhere—grocery stores, apps, drive-thrus—and our innate guidance system struggles to keep up. In this world of abundance, these natural signals are often overridden. You're no longer eating because you're hungry; you're eating because it's there, or because a commercial made that burger look irresistible.

And here's the kicker: our modern lifestyles are disrupting this finely-tuned system. Lack of sleep, chronic stress, and poor eating habits all mess with the balance between ghrelin and leptin. Imagine this: you're running on four hours of sleep, grabbing whatever snack is closest to keep going. Your ghrelin skyrockets, screaming, "I'm starving!" while leptin, tired and overwhelmed, can barely whisper, "You've had enough." Over time, this imbalance can lead to hormone resistance, where your body no longer recognizes these signals correctly. The result? Eating more than you need, feeling unsatisfied even after meals, and struggling with weight gain.

THE DIET DILEMMA: SHORT-TERM WINS, LONG-TERM CHALLENGES

Here's where restrictive diets come into play. Popular trends like fasting, keto, and low-carb diets often feel revolutionary at first. They shock your system—drastically reducing calories or eliminating food groups—and your body responds by quickly burning stored fat, leading to rapid weight loss. It's exciting, right? The scale drops, and you feel like you've found the answer.

But here's the catch: while these diets work well initially, they often disrupt your homeostatic signals further in the long run. Drastic calorie cuts or carb eliminations send your body into "survival mode," slowing your metabolism and making your hunger hormones go haywire. Leptin levels drop, making it harder to feel full, while ghrelin levels rise, intensifying cravings. This sets the stage for binge eating and weight regain, trapping you in the infamous yo-yo dieting cycle.

It's not just about discipline or willpower—it's biology. Your body is fighting to restore balance, often pushing you to overeat after restrictive periods. The key to long-term success isn't shocking your system but working with it—nourishing your body in a way that aligns with its natural rhythm.

By understanding how our innate guidance system works, we can stop battling our bodies and start listening to them. After all, your body isn't your enemy; it's just trying to help you survive. The challenge in today's world is learning how to honor those signals again and create an environment where they can work as they were designed.

THE LONG-TERM REALITY OF RESTRICTIVE DIETS

Yes, cutting carbs and increasing fat through diets like keto can initially work wonders for suppressing hunger hormones like ghrelin, making you feel less hungry. The increased fat intake provides a slow-burning energy source and helps you feel fuller for longer, creating that initial sense of control and success. At first, it feels like you've hacked the system, but over time, your body begins to push back. It starts sending signals that it's being deprived of essential nutrients, even if you're eating "healthy" foods like leafy greens, avocados, and fatty fish.

The truth is, restrictive diets often leave out vital nutrients found in fruits, legumes, and whole grains—like fiber, potassium, magnesium, and vitamin C. Without these, your body's functioning can falter, leading to side effects like digestive issues, fatigue, muscle cramps, and the ever-unwelcome companion: constipation.

Some may say, "But I'm eating nutrient-rich foods!" And that's valid—keto or low-carb diets can include great choices like nuts, seeds, and vegetables. The problem arises when meals lack variety and balance. Over-relying on high-fat options like meats, cheeses, or processed keto-friendly products while cutting out nutrient-dense foods like whole grains and certain fruits can still lead to deficiencies, even with otherwise "healthy" meals. It's not just about what you're eating—it's about what's missing.

THE MENTAL AND EMOTIONAL TOLL OF NUTRIENT DEPRIVATION

Then, there's the mental and emotional cost. When your body doesn't get enough nutrients, it reacts by amplifying hunger signals. What started as a diet that left you feeling empowered can quickly shift to a constant battle against hunger. You might find yourself irritable, foggy-headed, and battling the infamous hanger (hunger-induced anger). These intensified cravings make it harder to stick to the plan.

Eventually, your body's natural survival instincts take over. Deprivation triggers a biological response, making you more likely to overeat or binge on the very foods you've been trying to avoid. This cycle doesn't just undermine your progress—it can leave you feeling defeated, questioning your willpower, and stuck in the frustrating yo-yo of weight loss and regain.

A BALANCED APPROACH OVER RESTRICTION

Here's the truth: restrictive diets might give you quick results, but they rarely last. The constant cycle of deprivation can leave you feeling hungry, frustrated, and disconnected from your body. Instead of focusing on what you can't eat, why not shift your mindset to what you can add to your plate for balance? Think fiber-rich whole grains, colorful fruits, and nutrient-packed legumes—foods that not only nourish your body but also work with your natural signals, not against them.

The goal isn't just weight loss—it's building a lifestyle that supports your body, mind, and soul. When you prioritize balance over restriction, you're not just making temporary diet changes; you're laying the foundation for lasting health and happiness. And this is where a more intuitive approach comes in.

THE POWER OF INTUITIVE EATING

Intuitive eating is more than a trend—it's a powerful alternative to restrictive diets. Instead of following rigid rules or cutting out entire food groups, it encourages you to tune into your body's natural hunger and fullness cues. It's about eating when you're truly hungry and stopping when you're satisfied—no guilt, no restriction, no endless counting. This mindset helps rebuild the trust between your mind and body that restrictive diets often erode.

Let's break it down with a real-life example. Imagine you're at a family gathering, faced with a feast of your favorite dishes. As you savor your meal, you notice your body signaling that you're full. Instead of continuing to eat out of habit or fear of missing out, you pause and honor that fullness. Now, flip the scenario. You're feeling hungry between meals but decide to "power through" because your diet plan says snacks are off-limits. Intuitive eating challenges this rigid thinking. It encourages you to listen to your body's needs and nourish it when it asks—without guilt or second-guessing.

RECONNECTING WITH YOUR BODY'S NATURAL CUES

When we constantly ignore our hunger and fullness signals—whether by overeating or under-eating—we lose touch with our body's innate ability to regulate itself. Intuitive eating invites you to reconnect with these signals, helping you avoid extremes of deprivation or overindulgence. It's not about achieving perfection but about fostering trust: trust that your body knows what it needs and trust in your ability to respond mindfully.

This approach isn't just about food—it's about mindset. And when it comes to sustainable weight loss and overall well-being, mindset is everything. Intuitive eating shifts the focus from external rules to internal awareness, creating a healthier and more balanced relationship.

MINDSET: THE HIDDEN FORCE BEHIND WEIGHT LOSS

Let's talk about the real powerhouse behind lasting weight loss: your mindset.

We've all had those moments—the inner dialogue that whispers, "It's just one snack," or "I'll start fresh tomorrow." While these thoughts may seem harmless, they often grow into habits that hold us back. The truth is, the stories we tell ourselves about food shape our actions. If we don't address the mental and emotional roadblocks standing in our way, weight loss will always feel like an uphill battle.

Think of it this way: trying to lose weight while battling an inner voice that encourages indulgence is like driving with one foot on the gas and the other on the brake. Sure, you'll move forward, but it's slow, frustrating, and draining. The key to overcoming this struggle? Consistency and discipline. But here's the thing—discipline doesn't mean deprivation. It's about creating a mindset that keeps you motivated for the long haul, focusing on long-term health rather than fleeting satisfaction.

Your mindset is the driver behind the wheel, steering every decision you make. When you embrace the belief that maintaining a healthy weight leads to a better quality of life—more energy, better health, and greater confidence—it becomes easier to make choices that align with your goals, even in the face of temptation.

Humor can be your secret weapon here. Imagine the internal debate we've all had: "Should I grab that second slice of cake?" Instead of stressing over it, laugh at that little voice, acknowledge it, and confidently make the smarter choice. Life isn't about rigid rules—it's about balance, enjoying the journey, and letting go of guilt. You're in control here.

Part of shifting your mindset is reframing how you think about food. Instead of saying, "I can't have this," try saying, "I choose not to have this because it doesn't support my goals." That small mental shift puts you back in the driver's seat, turning food choices into empowering decisions rather than restrictions.

Remember, your mindset isn't just a passenger—it's the engine driving you forward. When you're clear on your why—whether it's better health, more energy, or simply feeling good in your own skin—staying committed to your goals becomes second nature. And when your mindset is aligned with your aspirations, everything else—consistency, discipline, and even those tough choices—falls into place.

EXERCISE AND GHRELIN: HOW MOVEMENT TAMES THE HUNGER HORMONE

Exercise is often hailed as a calorie-burning hero, but its impact on hormones—especially ghrelin, the "hunger hormone"—deserves just as much applause. Ghrelin signals your brain when it's time to eat, but here's the fascinating part: when you exercise, your body temperature rises, and ghrelin levels drop. That's why, after a good workout, you might find yourself less hungry, even though you've just burned energy.

It's like exercise flips a hormonal switch that helps keep your appetite in check.

But the benefits don't stop there. Exercise does so much more than curb hunger. It boosts your mood, strengthens your muscles (hello, metabolism!), and makes long-term weight management more achievable. And here's the best part: it doesn't have to be grueling or time-consuming. Just 10-20 minutes of daily movement—whether it's a brisk walk, a calming yoga session, or a quick bodyweight workout—can work wonders for your body and mind.

The key is finding something you genuinely enjoy. When movement becomes a joyful, natural part of your routine, it stops feeling like a chore and starts feeling like self-care. So lace up those sneakers, roll out that yoga mat, or dance around your living room—your hormones, metabolism, and mood will thank you.

GUT HEALTH: THE SECRET KEY TO WEIGHT LOSS

Your gut is home to trillions of bacteria, and their balance—specifically the ratio of Firmicutes to Bacteroidetes—plays a surprisingly powerful role in your weight and overall health. Let's break it down in relatable terms: think of Firmicutes as the "calorie hoarders" and Bacteroidetes as the "calorie sharers." Firmicutes are really efficient at extracting energy from food, which sounds great—until it leads to weight gain because your body absorbs more calories than it needs. On the other hand, Bacteroidetes are more laid-back, letting you burn energy more freely and helping to maintain a healthier weight.

When your gut has too many Firmicutes relative to Bacteroidetes, it's like your body is holding onto every last calorie from that delicious pasta dinner, making it harder to lose weight. But when this balance shifts toward more Bacteroidetes, your metabolism works more efficiently, supporting weight loss and reducing inflammation.

So, how do you keep your gut in check? Start by feeding your gut bacteria what they love: probiotics (like yogurt, kombucha, and sauerkraut) to introduce good bacteria, and prebiotics (like oats, bananas, and garlic) to nourish them. It's like hosting a party for the bacteria that help your metabolism thrive while giving the unhelpful ones less to work with.

The best part? This isn't about another restrictive diet—it's about small, sustainable changes that make you feel good from the inside out. By focusing on your gut health, you're not just improving digestion; you're boosting your body's ability to manage weight naturally. Think of your gut as your secret ally—nurture it, and it'll have your back on your weight loss journey.

THE JOURNEY TO SUSTAINABLE WEIGHT LOSS

Weight loss isn't about quick fixes or temporary solutions—it's a marathon, not a sprint. Crash diets might give you fast results, but they're often short-lived, leaving you frustrated and back where you started. Instead of chasing rapid weight loss, focus on building small, consistent habits that will carry you for a lifetime.

Set realistic goals, like losing 1-2 pounds a week rather than 10 pounds in a month. This slow and steady approach keeps your metabolism humming and avoids the rebound effect of extreme measures. Start with simple changes, like swapping sugary snacks for nuts, fruit, or Greek yogurt. Find movement you enjoy—a brisk 10-minute walk after dinner, a quick stretch in the morning, or dancing around the house with your kids.

Creating a flexible routine is key. Life isn't perfect, and neither is your journey. Allow room for the occasional indulgence without guilt. Enjoy a slice of cake at a celebration or a dinner out with friends—it's part of living a balanced life. Sustainable weight loss comes from building a lifestyle you love, not one you dread.

Most importantly, remember this: it's about progress, not perfection. Each small step forward, each choice to nourish your body, brings you closer to your goals. Celebrate those wins, no matter how small, because they're the foundation of lasting success. Weight loss isn't just about the number on the scale—it's about reclaiming your health, your energy, and your confidence, one step at a time.

STRATEGIES FOR MINDFUL EATING

The way you eat matters just as much as what's on your plate. Mindful eating is about being fully present during meals, helping you listen to your body's natural hunger and fullness signals. By eating more consciously, you can avoid overeating and develop a healthier relationship with food. Here's how to get started:

Cook More Meals at Home: Preparing your own meals lets you control ingredients and portion sizes. Plus, cooking can be a relaxing, creative activity that connects you to your food. If your schedule is hectic, aim for healthier options when dining out—choose dishes packed with lean proteins, whole grains, and vibrant veggies.

Eliminate Distractions: Ever polished off an entire bag of chips while watching TV? It's easy to lose track of how much you're eating when your attention is elsewhere. Turn off the screens and focus on your plate. Savor each bite, notice the flavors, and enjoy the experience of eating.

Slow Down: Your stomach needs time to signal your brain that it's full—usually about 20 minutes. Eating too quickly can lead to overeating before your body catches up. Take smaller bites, chew thoroughly, and pause between bites to truly enjoy your meal.

Serve Balanced Portions: Start with smaller portions and go back for seconds if you're still hungry. This prevents overloading your plate and encourages you to assess your hunger as you eat.

Listen to Your Body: Before reaching for seconds or a snack, ask yourself: Am I truly hungry, or am I eating out of boredom, stress, or habit? Honoring your body's cues helps you eat only when you're genuinely hungry.

Incorporating these mindful eating practices isn't just about weight loss—it's about fostering a healthy, balanced relationship with food. When you treat meals as intentional moments, you'll feel more satisfied, in control, and connected to your body.

RELAXATION AND STRESS MANAGEMENT: A KEY TO WEIGHT LOSS

Stress often flies under the radar as a major contributor to weight gain. When you're stressed, your body releases cortisol, a hormone that not only spikes cravings for sugary, high-fat comfort foods but also signals your body to store fat—especially around your midsection. This stress-induced fat storage can be a significant barrier to weight loss.

The solution? Build relaxation into your routine. Practices like yoga, meditation, deep breathing, or even taking a calming walk in nature can lower cortisol levels and help you manage stress effectively. These moments of relaxation are not indulgences—they are vital for both your mental and physical well-being. By keeping stress in check, you're not just protecting your peace of mind; you're also setting the stage for successful, sustainable weight loss.

SLEEP: THE SECRET WEAPON FOR WEIGHT LOSS SUCCESS

Sleep is often overlooked in weight loss discussions, but it's a game-changer. A lack of quality sleep can throw your hunger hormones into chaos. When you're sleep-deprived, ghrelin—the hormone that tells your brain you're hungry—goes into overdrive, while leptin—the hormone that signals you're full—drops. This imbalance creates a perfect storm for overeating.

Add to that the fatigue that comes from too little sleep, and it's no surprise that you reach for sugary, high-calorie snacks to keep going. Unfortunately, this sets off a vicious cycle of poor sleep and unhealthy eating habits, ultimately leading to weight gain.

Prioritize getting 7-9 hours of quality sleep each night to restore balance to your hunger hormones and keep your energy levels steady. Think of sleep as a vital component of your weight loss plan—it helps you recharge, reduces cravings, and keeps your body operating at its best. By making rest a priority, you're investing in a healthier, happier you.

CONCLUSION: EMBRACE THE JOURNEY TO LIFELONG HEALTH

This journey isn't about quick fixes or magic solutions—it's about choosing yourself every single day and building a life that nourishes your body, mind, and spirit. Your worth is not tied to a number on the scale or the size of your jeans; it's reflected in the love, care, and effort you give to yourself. Weight loss is not about deprivation—it's about reclaiming your health, confidence, and joy.

Every small step you take matters. Whether it's swapping out processed snacks for whole foods, committing to that 10-minute walk, or silencing the inner critic that tells you "you can't," these moments add up to something powerful. This isn't a sprint; it's a marathon fueled by consistency, self-compassion, and resilience.

Yes, there will be days when you feel stuck, unmotivated, or like you've taken a step back. That's okay. Setbacks are part of the process, not the end of the story. What defines you is your decision to rise, to keep moving forward, and to celebrate every win —big or small.

You already have what it takes to succeed. Start with one small change today. Whether it's drinking an extra glass of water, packing a balanced lunch, or setting aside 15 minutes for self-care, these actions signal to your body and mind that you're committed. Listen to what your body needs, honor its signals, and remind yourself daily: you are worth the effort.

The life you dream of—the energy, confidence, and health—is within your reach. Embrace this moment as a fresh start. Take control of your narrative and create the vibrant, fulfilling future you deserve. You've got this.

CHAPTER 14

HOLISTIC SKINCARE: A LOVE LETTER TO YOUR SKIN

THE ULTIMATE GUIDE TO AGELESS, NATURALLY RADIANT SKIN

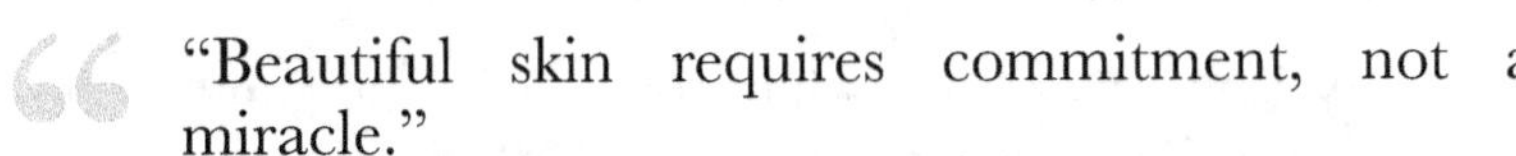

"Beautiful skin requires commitment, not a miracle."

— Erno Laszlo.

DO YOU LOVE YOUR SKIN?

Before you answer, "Of course, I do!" take a moment to think about it. Imagine your skin as a close friend—someone who mirrors your internal and external health. Would this "skin-friend" describe you as a caring, attentive companion, or someone who only shows up when there's a problem?

Let me tell you about my friend, Sarah. She had always been proud of her smooth complexion, but over a few months, her skin began to look unusually pale and dull. She tried every cream and serum she could find, but nothing worked. Concerned, she finally visited her doctor, who discovered she was severely anemic. Her skin wasn't just calling for attention—it was crying out for help. Once Sarah started addressing her anemia with the right nutrients, her skin transformed. It was a powerful reminder that our skin is often the first to show us when something's off inside.

Holistic skincare is about more than slathering on creams or following the latest beauty trend. It's an intimate partnership between you and your body, reflecting how you nourish yourself —inside and out. Your skin is a storyteller, revealing your stress levels, nutrition, hydration, and even your sleep patterns. So, how do you achieve radiant, healthy skin through a holistic approach?

This chapter is your guide to building a skincare routine that doesn't just treat the surface but embraces the full picture— body, mind, and spirit. Let's dive into how you can transform your relationship with your skin and let your natural beauty shine through.

WHAT IS HOLISTIC SKINCARE?

True beauty isn't just about what you see in the mirror—it's about how you feel in your own skin. Holistic skincare takes beauty beyond the surface, focusing on the powerful connection between your mind, body, and environment. Your skin is a reflection of your lifestyle, and the choices you make every day —what you eat, how you handle stress, and how you care for yourself—leave their mark.

Think about it: our skin is exposed to a constant barrage of stressors—pollution, UV rays, hormonal fluctuations, and even the blue light from our screens. These challenges can leave our skin dull, tired, and crying out for help. That's where holistic skincare shines. Instead of just masking surface-level concerns with quick fixes, it digs deeper, addressing the root causes. Whether the culprit is poor nutrition, stress, or daily habits, a holistic approach encourages you to heal your skin from the inside out.

Holistic skincare isn't just about creams and serums—it's a mindset. It's about understanding that what you put into your body, and even what you take away (like processed foods or toxic habits), affects your radiance. Think of it as giving your skin a daily love letter filled with healthy ingredients, mindful care, and a dash of patience.

Yes, this approach takes time and effort—no overnight miracles here—but the rewards are worth it. Holistic skincare is about transforming not just your skin, but your overall health and confidence. When you embrace this approach, you're not just caring for your skin—you're nurturing the vibrant, beautiful woman within.

Let's dive into how holistic skincare can help you glow, inside and out.

HOLISTIC SKINCARE: IT'S ALL CONNECTED!

Holistic skincare begins with a simple yet powerful truth: **your body is a beautifully interconnected system**. What happens inside reflects on the outside, and addressing one area often has a ripple effect across your entire well-being. This isn't about chasing the next trendy cream or indulging in Instagram-worthy face masks (though they're fun). It's about taking a whole-body approach that nurtures your health, your habits, and yes, your happiness.

Here's the glow-up secret: **when you enrich every part of your life, your skin will shine like never before.** A healthy lifestyle is the foundation of radiant skin—it's the behind-the-scenes magic that no product can replace. Think of your daily skincare routine as your skin's love language. And no, this doesn't mean you need to adopt a 10-step process. Seriously, who has time to feel like they're auditioning for a skincare commercial every morning?

Instead, simplicity is key. A consistent morning and night routine—cleanse, moisturize, protect—can work wonders. Your skin doesn't need to be pampered like royalty every day (although it wouldn't hurt occasionally), but it does appreciate thoughtful attention. Treat it well, and it will thank you with that lit-from-within glow.

So, whether it's starting your day with a splash of cold water or winding down with a nourishing moisturizer, remember this: **you don't need perfection—you need consistency.** Just like brushing your teeth or making that essential cup of morning coffee, your skincare routine is a non-negotiable habit. Let's dive into how you can simplify, connect, and transform your skin from the inside out.

DEVELOPING A ROUTINE: WHAT SHOULD IT INCLUDE?

So, how do you even start building a skincare routine? Let me take you back to when my "routine" was more like an afterthought. I'd hurriedly wash my face before bed (on a good day), skip toner entirely, apply sunscreen only on sunny vacations, and scrub my face like I was trying to buff out a scratch on my car.

To make matters worse, I'd then collapse onto a cotton pillow-case that wasn't doing my skin any favors. The result? Redness, breakouts, and that stubborn rough texture that no amount of moisturizer seemed to fix. It didn't take long for me to realize that my so-called "routine" was actually part of the problem.

Lesson learned: **consistency matters, and so does how you treat your skin.** The goal is to care for your skin, not wage war on it. And while the pinky-and-ring-finger washing method sounds intriguing, let's be real—no one has the time or patience for a two-finger facial cleanse every night. So, here's what you really need to know about washing your face properly.

THE ART OF FACE WASHING: LESS PRESSURE, BETTER RESULTS

When it comes to washing your face, many of us assume that more pressure equals a deeper clean. But the truth? **Less is more.** The skin on your face is delicate, especially around the eyes, and excessive scrubbing can actually damage its elasticity and lead to premature aging. The key isn't in how hard you scrub but in how gently and thoroughly you cleanse.

How to Wash Your Face Like a Pro

1. **Use your fingertips:** Instead of scrubbing with your whole hand or palm, use your fingertips in gentle, circular motions. This technique ensures you're cleaning without pulling or stretching the skin.
2. **Lather up lightly:** Apply a dime-sized amount of cleanser and let it foam naturally—no need to go overboard. Choose a gentle cleanser that suits your skin type.
3. **Consider the spray effect:** If you're looking for an even gentler option, think about using the spray from your shower or a faucet. The soft water stream acts as a natural cleanser, loosening dirt and oil without requiring any pressure from your hands. Just make sure the water is lukewarm to avoid drying out your skin.
4. **Focus on problem areas:** Pay extra attention to spots like the T-zone (forehead, nose, and chin), where oil and dirt tend to build up. But don't forget the jawline and hairline, which often get neglected.
5. **Rinse thoroughly:** Whether you use a spray or your hands, make sure to rinse your face completely. Residual cleanser can lead to irritation, so take your time to wash it all away.
6. **Pat, don't rub:** Use a clean, soft towel to pat your face dry. Rubbing can irritate the skin and undo all your gentle cleansing work.

By adopting these simple techniques, you're not just washing your face—you're creating a routine that protects and nurtures your skin over time. Remember, **your skin appreciates the love you show it** through thoughtful, gentle care. A proper cleanse is the first step toward a radiant, glowing complexion.

HOLISTIC LIFESTYLE AND YOUR SKIN: MORE THAN SKIN-DEEP

Did you know your skin is the largest organ in your body? That's right—it's like the overachiever in your anatomy, doing way more than just keeping you looking fabulous. Your skin acts as your body's first line of defense, blocking harmful microbes, toxins, and pollutants while locking in all the good stuff—like moisture and nutrients. It's also your personal thermostat, keeping you cool when you're overheating and cozy when it's chilly. Oh, and it's a multitasking genius, aiding in vitamin D production while being packed with nerve endings that help you feel everything from a soft breeze to that dreaded accidental brush against a hot curling iron. Ouch!

Ever notice how your skin seems to glow after a full night of glorious, uninterrupted sleep? Or how a stressful week has the uncanny ability to summon a breakout that feels like it needs its own zip code? That's the skin-body connection at work.

By making small, intentional changes to your daily habits—like eating nutrient-rich foods, hydrating, managing stress, and catching those z's—you're not just improving your skin. You're improving your whole self. When your body is happy, your skin becomes the glowing billboard announcing it to the world. After all, your skin is working overtime to keep you looking and feeling your best!

THE IMPORTANCE OF KNOWING YOUR SKIN TYPE

Let's be real—taking care of your skin without knowing its type is like trying to solve a puzzle with missing pieces. The way your skin behaves impacts everything from your product choices to your routine. There are four main skin types: **normal, dry, oily, and combination.** If you're unsure about yours, no problem—let's figure it out together.

Normal Skin: The Gold Standard

If you have normal skin, congratulations! You've hit the skincare jackpot. Normal skin is well-balanced—neither too oily nor too dry. You probably don't deal with pesky breakouts or flaky patches often, but that doesn't mean you can slack off. Regular cleansing, moisturizing, and sunscreen are still must-haves to maintain that natural glow. Think of it as preventive maintenance for your already happy skin.

Dry Skin: Hydration Is Your Best Friend

Dry skin often feels tight, rough, or itchy, especially after cleansing. It's thirsty—craving hydration like a plant in a desert. If this sounds familiar, your first line of defense is a rich moisturizer and a gentle cleanser that won't strip your skin's natural oils. Pro tip: adding a humidifier to your home can help restore moisture to your skin, especially in colder months. Your skin will thank you with a softer, more supple feel.

Oily Skin: Shine Bright, But Not Too Bright

Oily skin has a way of making its presence known—shiny T-zone, clogged pores, and breakouts, anyone? But here's the thing: oily skin isn't your enemy; it just needs the right TLC. Wash your face twice a day with a gentle cleanser, keep blotting papers handy, and always moisturize with an **oil-free, lightweight moisturizer.** Yes, oily skin needs hydration too, or it might overcompensate and produce even more oil. Think of it as a truce with your skin—you hydrate it right, and it won't rebel.

Combination Skin: A Little Bit of Everything

Combination skin is like a mood swing—it can't decide between oily or dry. The T-zone (forehead, nose, chin) often resembles an oil slick, while the cheeks can feel as dry as the

Sahara. The key to managing combination skin is **targeted care**: use a toner or lightweight moisturizer for oily areas and a richer cream for the dry spots. Treating each area like it has its own personality is the secret to harmony.

MY JOURNEY WITH COMBINATION SKIN

I get it—managing combination skin can feel like juggling two skincare routines at once. Back in the day, I didn't realize my oily T-zone and dry cheeks needed different treatments. I'd slap on the same moisturizer everywhere and wonder why my nose shined brighter than a disco ball while my cheeks looked parched.

Now, I've cracked the code. A lightweight, water-based moisturizer for my T-zone and a richer, creamy one for my cheeks have made all the difference. I've even introduced products with **hyaluronic acid** to hydrate without making my skin greasy. Balance isn't just the key to life—it's also the secret to glowing skin.

ZOOMING IN: OILY SKIN'S T-ZONE TROUBLE

For those with oily skin, it's usually the **T-zone** that takes the spotlight. This area, spanning the forehead, nose, and chin, tends to produce more oil than the rest of the face. If you've ever looked in the mirror and felt like your nose was auditioning to be a mirror ball at a party, you're not alone. The good news? With the right products and a consistent routine, you can keep that shine in check while letting your natural glow shine through.

WHY KNOWING YOUR SKIN TYPE MATTERS

Understanding your skin type isn't just a beauty hack—it's the foundation of effective skincare. It saves you from wasting money on products that don't work and ensures your routine is tailored to what your skin truly needs. So, take a moment, evaluate your skin, and start treating it with the love and care it deserves. Because when your skin feels good, you feel good. And that, my friend, is a glow no highlighter can match.

GLOW FROM WITHIN: THE HOLISTIC APPROACH TO RADIANT SKIN

Ready to achieve that enviable, radiant glow? Let's explore some lifestyle habits that not only transform your skin but also nurture your overall well-being. Holistic care isn't just a trendy term—it's the foundation for healthy, vibrant skin.

As a nurse, I've witnessed firsthand how neglecting self-care—whether through poor diets, chronic stress, or sleep deprivation—can take a toll. And where does it often show up first? Right on your face. Wrinkles, dullness, breakouts—they're like your skin's way of waving a red flag.

Your body is like a finely-tuned machine, and the better you care for it, the more it rewards you. Let's dive into the skin-loving habits that will help you radiate from the inside out.

EAT YOUR WAY TO RADIANT SKIN: SKIN-LOVING FOODS YOU'LL ACTUALLY ENJOY

We've all heard the phrase, "You are what you eat," but when it comes to your skin, it's not just a catchy saying—it's science. Your skin mirrors what's happening on the inside, and a nutrient-rich diet can work wonders for that coveted glow. On the flip side, poor food choices can lead to dullness, breakouts, or even flare-ups of stubborn skin conditions. Let's dive into the grocery list that your skin will thank you for:

The Skin-Loving Superstars:

- **Coconut Oil**: Sure, it's a kitchen staple, but coconut oil is like a multitasking skincare MVP. Packed with fatty acids, it nourishes and protects your skin while reducing inflammation. Pro tip: dab a little on dry patches—it works wonders!

- **Avocados**: These creamy gems aren't just Instagram-worthy—they're loaded with vitamins, minerals, and healthy fats that keep your skin soft, supple, and radiant. Think of avocados as nature's moisturizer that works from the inside out.
- **Tomatoes**: Who knew your salad could double as sun protection? Tomatoes are rich in lycopene, an antioxidant that helps guard against UV damage and inflammation. So, yes, eating tomatoes is basically sunscreen you can snack on.
- **Green Tea**: Swap your afternoon coffee for green tea and sip your way to calmer skin. Its anti-inflammatory properties help reduce redness, and antioxidants fight free radicals that age your skin. Plus, it's hydrating—win-win!
- **Sweet Potatoes**: These vibrant root veggies are packed with beta-carotene, which your body converts to vitamin A. That's the magic vitamin for repairing and generating new skin cells. Say hello to a smoother complexion!
- **Blueberries**: Don't underestimate these tiny fruits—they're loaded with antioxidants like anthocyanins, which protect your skin from environmental damage. And with their vitamin C and E content, they're collagen-boosters in disguise.

RICE WATER: YOUR KITCHEN BEAUTY SECRET

Now for a little curveball: rice water. Nope, you're not eating it (though, no judgment if you do). This humble byproduct of cooking rice is a powerhouse for your skin. Packed with vitamins B and C, plus skin-friendly minerals like magnesium and potassium, rice water is like the underdog beauty hack you didn't know you needed.

Why rice water rocks: It's full of antioxidants that combat aging and reduce elastase activity—the enzyme responsible for making your skin lose elasticity. Translation? It's basically a DIY youth elixir straight from your kitchen.

How to use it:

1. Save the leftover water from your cooked rice (preferably organic, because your skin deserves the best).
2. After cleansing, apply it to your face with a cotton ball.
3. Let it sit for 10–15 minutes, then rinse off. Think of it as a spa treatment without the hefty price tag. Your skin will look so refreshed that people might ask where you've been vacationing.

REAL TALK: MAKE IT SUSTAINABLE

While these foods can transform your skin, consistency is key. You don't need a complete pantry overhaul—start small. Add blueberries to your morning oatmeal, swap your snack for green tea, or drizzle a little coconut oil on your roasted sweet potatoes.

And hey, life's about balance. Indulge in your favorites every now and then—just remember, it's the everyday habits that build lasting change. After all, when you're glowing from within, it's not just your skin that shines—it's your confidence, too.

SUMMARIZING SLEEP AND SELF-CARE: BEAUTY REST IS NO MYTH

Let's start with a universal truth: *beauty sleep is real*. While you snooze, your body is hard at work repairing and regenerating cells, including those in your skin. Think of it as your personal overnight spa treatment—no fancy creams required. Those golden 7-9 hours of rest can be the secret to waking up with a fresher, brighter complexion. So, if you've been skimping on sleep, consider this your nudge to make bedtime a sacred ritual. Your skin (and mood) will thank you.

Simple Tips for Better Beauty Sleep:

- **Stick to a Schedule:**Going to bed and waking up at the same time daily helps regulate your internal clock.
- **Unplug Before Bed:**Swap late-night scrolling for a quick meditation or your favorite book.
- **Create a Cozy Vibe:**Keep your room cool, dark, and quiet—a little sanctuary for sweet dreams.

CHOOSING THE RIGHT INGREDIENTS FOR YOUR SKIN

Skincare isn't one-size-fits-all, and the products you use matter just as much as the food you eat. Let's break down what to look for—and what to avoid—when curating your skin's menu. After all, your skin deserves the best, and understanding these ingredients is like reading the label on your favorite snack: essential for knowing what's good for you.

Skin-Loving Ingredients to Seek Out

- **Niacinamide (Vitamin B3):** Think of niacinamide as your skin's best multitasking friend. It strengthens the skin barrier, reduces large pores, brightens your complexion, and fights inflammation. Sensitive or acne-prone? Niacinamide's got your back (and face).
- **Zinc Oxide:** A powerhouse ingredient in sun protection, this mineral creates a physical barrier that reflects harmful UV rays. Unlike chemical sunscreens, it won't irritate sensitive skin. Daily use helps prevent premature aging, dark spots, and skin cancer— seriously, wear your sunscreen.
- **Lutein:** The anti-blue light warrior. If you're glued to screens all day (who isn't?), lutein helps protect your

skin from blue light's sneaky aging effects. Found in green veggies, it's like armor for your skin.

- **Hyaluronic Acid:** Dry skin? Hyaluronic acid is like a tall glass of water for your face. It locks in moisture, giving you that plump, dewy glow without clogging pores.
- **Vitamin C:** This powerhouse brightens skin, reduces dark spots, and boosts collagen for a youthful look. If hyperpigmentation or dullness is your nemesis, Vitamin C is your superhero.
- **Ceramides:** Think of ceramides as your skin's glue. They help form the barrier that locks in moisture and keeps irritants out. If your skin feels dry or irritated, it's likely crying out for more ceramides.
- **Peptides:** These little building blocks work to firm your skin and smooth out fine lines. It's like giving your skin a pep talk to repair and rejuvenate itself.

Ingredients to Avoid (For the Sake of Your Skin and Sanity)

- **Parabens:** Linked to hormone disruption, these preservatives are best avoided. Opt for products labeled "paraben-free" to stay on the safe side.
- **Sulfates:** Sure, they create a satisfying lather, but they strip away your skin's natural oils. If your face feels tight after cleansing, sulfates might be to blame.
- **Phthalates:** Often hiding under the label "fragrance" or "parfum," these can mess with your hormones. Choose fragrance-free products instead.
- **Alcohol (Denatured, Isopropyl):** These harsh alcohols dry out your skin and speed up aging. Your skin deserves better than a product that feels like paint thinner.
- **Triclosan:** Found in antibacterial soaps, this ingredient disrupts hormones and encourages antibiotic-resistant bacteria. Plus, it's terrible for the environment—double no.

- **Oxybenzone:** A common sunscreen ingredient that harms coral reefs and disrupts hormones. Look for "reef-safe" sunscreens to protect both your skin and the planet.

MAKING SKINCARE RELATABLE (AND A BIT FUN)

Think of skincare like grocery shopping—you wouldn't toss an unpronounceable, suspicious ingredient into your cart, so why do it with your skincare? Just as you'd choose ripe avocados over a bruised, sad one at the store, the same goes for your skincare products. Quality always wins over quantity. The right ingredients nourish your skin, while the wrong ones can leave it pleading for mercy.

And let's not forget the self-care angle. Treating your skin well isn't just about avoiding wrinkles or banishing breakouts; it's about creating a routine that feels good and works for you. Whether it's indulging in a Vitamin C serum or saying goodbye to that harsh cleanser, every little choice adds up to a happier, healthier you.

When you're selecting skincare products, think of it as an investment—not just in today's glow but in the long-term health of your skin. Ingredients like niacinamide, zinc oxide, and lutein work together to protect, hydrate, and rejuvenate. On the flip side, harmful additives like parabens, sulfates, and phthalates can wreak havoc.

So, next time you're skincare shopping, don't just reach for the prettiest bottle on the shelf. Take a moment to check the ingredients, make informed choices, and choose products that truly serve your skin's needs. Trust me, your skin—and future you—will thank you for it. Now go ahead and give your skin the love it deserves. You're already glowing!

NOURISHING YOUR SKIN FROM THE INSIDE OUT WITH VITAMINS AND WATER:

We all dream of that effortless, radiant glow that says, *"I'm totally thriving—yes, I get 8 hours of sleep, eat like a wellness guru, and never miss leg day."* But let's be honest—real life doesn't always look like that. Between chaotic schedules, late-night snacks, and that third cup of coffee, our skin can sometimes feel like it's waving a white flag.

Here's the good news: even when life gets messy, there are practical ways to nourish your skin from the inside out. Vitamins, hydration, and quality sleep are your skin's three best friends. Let's break them down into doable steps that fit into your real-life routine. Bonus: no kale obsession required (unless you're into that).

Daily Supplements: Little Boosts, Big Beauty Wins

Let's face it—eating a rainbow of veggies every day sounds amazing, but sometimes it's more like *pizza with a side of fries.* That's where supplements come in. They're like your skin's safety net, giving it what it needs when life gets hectic.

- **Vitamin A:** This skin superhero promotes cell turnover, keeps your skin hydrated, and smooths fine lines. Think carrots, leafy greens, and sweet potatoes—or grab a supplement if "eating the garden" isn't your vibe.
- **Vitamin C:** The glow-getter of the group! It brightens your skin, boosts collagen, and fights free radicals. Citrus fruits, strawberries, and bell peppers are great sources, but a morning Vitamin C tablet works wonders too (especially for the coffee-and-toast crowd).
- **Omega-3 Fatty Acids:** These healthy fats keep your skin plump and hydrated. You'll find them in salmon,

chia seeds, and flaxseed oil—or take a capsule if you're not into fishy flavors.

- **Biotin & Collagen:**Think of these as reinforcements for your skin, hair, and nails. They strengthen your skin's resilience, helping it look and feel its best.

Remember, supplements aren't magic potions. They're part of a team effort, working alongside your diet and habits to keep your skin happy.

ELIMINATE THE BAD FROM YOUR LIFE: WHY IT MATTERS FOR YOUR SKIN

Achieving good skin isn't just about finding the perfect serum or moisturizer—it's about being mindful of what you consume and how it affects your body. Here's why some common habits and substances can wreak havoc on your skin, explained with science and actionable alternatives.

1. Sugar: The Silent Skin Saboteur

Sugar is infamous for being harmful to your skin, and here's why:

- **How Sugar Causes Inflammation:** When you consume sugar, your blood sugar levels spike, causing your body to release insulin. This triggers a cascade of inflammatory responses as your body tries to stabilize the sugar levels. Inflammation, in turn, affects your skin by breaking down **collagen** and **elastin**, the proteins responsible for keeping your skin firm, plump, and youthful. Over time, this leads to sagging skin and wrinkles.
- **Sugar and Breakouts:** Excess sugar fuels the growth of harmful bacteria in your gut and contributes to hormonal imbalances by increasing androgen production, which can lead to clogged pores and acne breakouts.

- **The Glycation Effect:** Sugar molecules attach to proteins in a process called glycation, forming harmful compounds known as **Advanced Glycation End Products (AGEs)**. These AGEs weaken skin structure, accelerate aging, and make your skin more vulnerable to environmental damage.
- **Alternative:** Swap sugary treats with naturally sweet fruits like berries, which are rich in antioxidants, or veggies like carrots and sweet potatoes. These provide sweetness while delivering vitamins that fight inflammation and oxidative stress.

2. Fried Food: Your Skin's Frenemy

We all love a crispy fry or golden fried chicken, but here's the hard truth: deep-fried foods are no friend to your skin. If you've read about how processed sugar can form **advanced glycation end products (AGEs)** and wreak havoc on your skin, guess what? Fried foods do the same thing—and they might even be worse.

The Science Behind the Damage

When foods are deep-fried at high temperatures, they undergo a process called **oxidation**, which leads to the formation of AGEs. These harmful compounds break down **collagen** and **elastin**, the proteins responsible for keeping your skin smooth, firm, and youthful. Over time, this leads to sagging, wrinkles, and a dull complexion.

The Role of Trans Fats and Free Radicals

Fried foods are often cooked in oils that degrade at high heat, generating **trans fats** and **free radicals**. Trans fats don't just harm your arteries—they also clog your pores, increasing the likelihood of acne and breakouts. Free radicals, on the other hand, cause **oxidative stress** in your skin cells, accelerating the aging process and leaving your skin more vulnerable to environmental damage.

Inflammation: The Real Culprit

Like sugar, fried foods promote **inflammation** in the body, which can exacerbate skin conditions like acne, eczema, and psoriasis. Inflammation also disrupts your skin barrier, making it harder for your skin to retain moisture and defend itself against irritants.

A Greasy Takeaway

While the occasional indulgence won't harm you, making fried foods a regular part of your diet can have long-term effects on your skin. Instead of reaching for fried chicken or fries, opt for healthier alternatives like baking, grilling, or air-frying. These methods can still give you that satisfying crunch without the skin-damaging side effects.

Your skin mirrors what you eat, and by cutting back on fried foods, you're giving your skin a chance to thrive. So, next time you're faced with a tempting plate of crispy fried goodness, remember: your skin deserves better!

3. Alcohol: Dehydration and Inflammation in a Glass

Alcohol may be fun in moderation, but your skin doesn't find it so amusing.

- **Dehydration and Its Effects on Skin:** Alcohol acts as a diuretic, pulling water out of your system. Dehydrated skin appears dull, flaky, and more prone to fine lines and wrinkles. Without adequate hydration, your skin's natural barrier weakens, leaving it vulnerable to damage and irritation.
- **Alcohol and Inflammation:** Alcohol increases inflammatory markers in the body, exacerbating skin conditions like acne, rosacea, and eczema. It can also cause facial redness and puffiness due to dilated blood vessels.
- **Alternative:** If you enjoy drinks, try non-alcoholic mocktails infused with antioxidant-rich ingredients like

lime, mint, or cucumber. Pair any alcohol consumption with plenty of water to reduce its dehydrating effects.

4. Cigarettes: Toxins That Steal Your Glow

Smoking is one of the worst habits for your skin, and here's why:

- **Free Radical Damage:** Cigarette smoke is loaded with toxins and free radicals that attack skin cells, breaking down collagen and elastin. This leads to premature wrinkles, sagging skin, and an overall dull complexion.
- **Reduced Blood Flow:** Smoking constricts blood vessels, limiting the oxygen and nutrient supply to your skin. The result? Your skin struggles to regenerate, leaving it looking lifeless and tired.
- **Delayed Healing:** Smokers experience slower wound healing due to reduced circulation, making skin more prone to scars and discoloration from acne or injuries.
- **Alternative:** If you smoke, quitting is the single best thing you can do for your skin and health. Seek support from a healthcare provider, nicotine replacement therapies, or counseling programs to make the process smoother.

WHY ELIMINATING THESE HABITS IS WORTH IT

When you cut out sugar, alcohol, and cigarettes, you're not just doing your skin a favor—you're transforming your entire body's health. Inflammation, dehydration, and oxidative stress are silent culprits that age your skin prematurely and lead to long-term damage. But by taking small, consistent steps to eliminate these bad habits, you'll not only see visible improvements in your skin but also feel more vibrant and energetic overall.

You don't have to do it all at once—start small. Skip dessert a couple of nights a week, opt for water instead of wine at dinner, or trade a cigarette break for a brisk walk. These changes add up to big results.

Your skin is your body's largest organ and its natural shield. Treat it with the love and care it deserves, and it will reflect your efforts with a healthy, radiant glow.

STRESS AND YOUR SKIN: WHY WE'RE TALKING ABOUT IT AGAIN

Yes, stress is a recurring topic in this book—and for good reason. Stress doesn't just impact your body and mind; it wreaks havoc on your skin. While we've explored stress management in earlier chapters, it's worth revisiting here with a focus on how stress directly affects your complexion. Why? Because understanding this connection empowers you to approach skincare holistically, tackling not just surface-level concerns but also the root causes.

Think of this as a deeper dive into why stress leaves its mark on your face—literally. From breakouts to premature aging, stress impacts your skin in ways you might not realize. While you've already learned tools to manage stress in other chapters, here we'll explore how reducing stress supports glowing, healthy skin. After all, managing stress isn't just about feeling good—it's about looking radiant, too.

HOW STRESS IMPACTS YOUR SKIN

When life gets overwhelming, your body releases cortisol, often referred to as the "stress hormone." While cortisol is helpful in short bursts, chronic stress keeps those cortisol levels elevated for too long. Here's what that does to your skin:

1. **Inflammation:** High cortisol levels trigger inflammation, which can worsen conditions like acne,

eczema, psoriasis, and rosacea. You might notice flare-ups happening right when you're already feeling frazzled.

2. **Collagen and Elastin Breakdown:** Cortisol also disrupts the production of collagen and elastin—your skin's natural scaffolding. This can lead to fine lines, wrinkles, and sagging skin, making stress a fast track to premature aging.

3. **Compromised Skin Barrier:** Stress can weaken your skin's protective barrier, leaving it more prone to dryness, irritation, and environmental damage.

4. **Oil Overload:** In response to stress, your skin may overproduce sebum (oil), leading to clogged pores and —you guessed it—breakouts.

Stress doesn't just show up on your face—it practically throws a party there. But the good news? You're the host, and you can shut it down.

REDUCING STRESS FOR BETTER SKIN: A QUICK REMINDER

You've probably read about stress management in the relaxation chapter, but it's worth emphasizing again—stress isn't just tough on your mind and body; it's a major culprit behind many skin issues. Managing stress is an essential part of any holistic skincare routine.

- **Carve out daily "me time."** Whether it's taking a quick walk outdoors, losing yourself in your favorite song in your personal sanctuary, or stepping away from social media to dive into a good book, even just 10 minutes can work wonders for both your stress levels and your skin.

- **Nourish and move your body.** Eating a balanced diet and staying active don't just help you feel good—they improve circulation, support skin repair, and keep your natural glow alive.

By embracing these small changes, you'll not only feel more balanced but also give your skin the love and care it deserves.

PAMPER YOURSELF: A LITTLE TLC GOES A LONG WAY

Looking good and feeling good go hand in hand. When your skin is glowing, you exude confidence, radiance, and that unmistakable *I've got it together* energy. But let's face it: sometimes, despite our best efforts, our skin doesn't look or feel its best. So how can you turn things around and give your skin the love it deserves? By indulging in a little pampering! Here are some simple yet powerful ways to revitalize your skin and your spirit.

Get a Facial (Or Create One at Home!)

Facials are a fantastic way to deeply cleanse, exfoliate, and rejuvenate your skin. They stimulate circulation, leaving you with that post-facial glow we all crave. While professional facials are amazing, they're not always budget- or schedule-friendly. The good news? You can create your own spa experience right at home! With a few simple steps and some DIY magic, you can give yourself a luxurious treatment that rivals the professionals.

Steps for Your Mini Home Spa

1. **Cleanse:** Start with a gentle, water-based cleanser to remove dirt, makeup, and impurities. This ensures your skin is clean but not stripped of its natural oils.
2. **Steam:** Steaming is like a warm hug for your pores. Use a bowl of hot water and drape a towel over your head to trap the steam, keeping a safe distance to avoid burns. This softens your skin and helps open your pores for deeper cleansing.
3. **Exfoliate:** Once your pores are open, use an exfoliant with alpha or beta hydroxy acids to slough away dead

skin cells. This step is crucial for revealing fresh, radiant skin beneath.

4. **Mask:** A good mask is your skin's best friend. Choose one tailored to your needs—hydrating, brightening, or detoxifying—and let it work its magic. Trust me, this is the step where your skin starts saying, "Thank you!"

5. **Serum:** After removing the mask, apply a serum like Vitamin C for brightening or retinol for anti-aging benefits. This step delivers concentrated nutrients directly to your skin.

6. **Massage:** Gently massage your face using upward strokes. This not only feels heavenly but also boosts circulation and promotes lymphatic drainage.

7. **Moisturize:** Lock in all that goodness with a hydrating moisturizer. This final step seals the deal, leaving your skin soft, plump, and glowing.

Masks and Serums: The Right Order for Maximum Benefit

The sequence of applying a mask and serum largely depends on the type of mask you're using and its purpose:

1. **Deep-Cleansing or Exfoliating Masks:** These masks, like clay masks or exfoliating masks, are designed to remove impurities, unclog pores, or exfoliate dead skin cells.
   - After the Mask: Your skin is now clean and primed, making it the perfect time to apply a serum. Serums are concentrated with active ingredients that penetrate deeply into your skin. Whether it's a Vitamin C serum for brightening or a hydrating hyaluronic acid serum, this step will lock in nourishment after the cleansing mask has done its job.

2. **Hydrating, Nourishing, or Sheet Masks:** Many nourishing masks, particularly sheet masks (like

Korean ones), are already soaked in a serum-like formula. These masks aim to deliver moisture, firm the skin, or rejuvenate with active ingredients.

- ○ After the Mask: In this case, you can often skip an additional serum because the mask itself has already infused your skin with active ingredients. Instead, gently pat the leftover serum from the mask into your skin to enhance absorption.
- ○ Optional Step: If your skin feels like it could benefit from an extra boost or if you have a specific serum you want to add (e.g., for anti-aging or acne), you can layer it on after the mask—but make sure it complements the ingredients already in the mask.

Here's a refined and engaging version of your content, designed to be clear, relatable, and motivational for your audience:

How to Choose the Right Ingredients for Your Facial Mask

Facial masks are like the cherry on top of your skincare routine—targeting specific concerns while giving your skin that much-needed TLC. With endless options on the market, from Amazon favorites to beloved Korean beauty gems, it's important to choose a mask tailored to your skin type and goals. Let's break it down:

1. Know Your Skin Type and Goals

Every skin type has its own unique needs, and the right mask can work wonders when matched correctly. Here's what to look for:

- **Dry Skin:** If your skin feels tight or flaky, go for masks with hydrating heroes like **hyaluronic acid**, **glycerin**, or **honey** to restore moisture and revitalize.

- **Oily or Acne-Prone Skin:** Struggling with shine or breakouts? Opt for ingredients like **clay**, **charcoal**, or **salicylic acid**, which absorb oil, unclog pores, and prevent future breakouts.
- **Sensitive Skin:** Gentle is the name of the game here. Look for calming ingredients like **oatmeal**, **chamomile**, or **cucumber extract** to reduce redness and soothe irritation.
- **Dull or Aging Skin:** If you're battling dullness or signs of aging, choose masks with **vitamin C**, **collagen**, or **peptides** to brighten, firm, and rejuvenate.
- **For Radiance and Brightening:** Unique ingredients like **snail mucin** or **gold particles** are popular in Korean skincare masks, offering hydration, skin repair, and anti-inflammatory effects.

Spotlight on Snail Mucin and Gold Particles

- **Snail Mucin**: It may sound unusual, but snail mucin is a skincare superstar. Packed with **hyaluronic acid**, **peptides**, and **glycolic acid**, it hydrates, repairs, and reduces signs of aging. Perfect for dry, scarred, or aging skin!
- **Gold Particles**: Add a touch of luxury to your routine. Gold helps brighten, calm inflammation, and stimulate collagen production for firmer, glowing skin.

2. Check the Label Like a Pro

Here's how to make sure you're getting the most out of your mask:

- **Natural Ingredients:**Fewer additives and chemicals are always better, especially for sensitive skin.
- **Ingredient Order:**Ingredients listed first are present in the highest amounts. Look for key actives like vitamin C or collagen at the top of the list.

- **Skin Type Recommendations:**Many masks specify if they're for dry, oily, or sensitive skin. Pay attention to avoid mismatches that could irritate your skin.
- **Popular Korean Ingredients:**Icons like **green tea**, **propolis**, and **ginseng** are known for their soothing, anti-aging, and brightening properties.

4. Make It a Ritual: Frequency and Self-Care

Using a facial mask 2-3 times a week can elevate your skincare routine and give you a moment of relaxation. Beyond skincare, this time can double as a mini self-care ritual—light a candle, put on your favorite music, and let the mask work its magic.

By understanding your skin's needs, checking the labels, and choosing the right mask, you're not just adding another step to your routine—you're investing in glowing, radiant skin. Because when your skin feels good, so do you!

PROTECT YOURSELF AGAINST SKIN DAMAGE

For quite some time, I didn't wear sunscreen. I thought I was embracing my "natural" side, but what I didn't realize was that my skin was bearing the brunt of UV exposure without any shield. It wasn't until a friend pointed out the brown spots on my face that I had my wake-up call. That's when I learned about the role of melanin in skin protection—and why sunscreen is so crucial.

When your skin is exposed to sunlight, it produces melanin, a natural pigment designed to shield your skin from the sun's harmful rays. Melanin acts as a defense mechanism by absorbing ultraviolet (UV) radiation, which helps prevent DNA damage in skin cells. However, when the skin is exposed repeatedly without protection, melanin production can go into overdrive, leading to visible brown spots or hyperpigmentation as a result of uneven melanin buildup.

But brown spots are only the beginning. With continued, unprotected exposure, the risk of DNA damage increases, which can lead to skin cancers, including melanoma. So, yes, those brown spots are a sign—and if we listen, they remind us that protection is essential for more than just cosmetic reasons.

If you're new to sunscreen, here's a reminder: SPF 30 or higher is your minimum, and it's essential to reapply every two hours, especially when swimming or sweating. Sunscreen, however, isn't the only part of the solution. The screens we use daily also emit harmful **blue light**, which penetrates deeply into the skin, accelerating aging and increasing pigmentation issues.

Here's how to manage both UV and blue light exposure:

1. **Apply Sunscreen Daily**: Choose a broad-spectrum sunscreen that covers both UVA and UVB rays. It's your first line of defense against aging and damage.
2. **Use Blue Light Filters on Devices**: Many smartphones and laptops now have "night mode" or "blue light filter" settings, which help reduce exposure. If possible, use these filters during screen time.
3. **Invest in Screen Protectors**: Look for screen protectors that filter out blue light. These are simple, effective, and can make a difference over time.
4. **Antioxidant-Rich Skincare**: Ingredients like niacinamide, lutein, and vitamin C help counteract free radical damage from blue light exposure, preserving your skin's elasticity and brightness.

SKIN CANCER AWARENESS: PROTECTING YOUR SKIN WITH A SMILE

When we talk about skincare, it's easy to focus on glowing skin, fewer wrinkles, and all the good stuff. But let's be real—healthy skin goes way beyond beauty products. One of the most important (and often overlooked) parts of a skincare routine is protection from skin cancer, a very preventable but potentially serious condition.

A friend of mine recently shared her journey with skin cancer, and her story made me pause and think. It all started with a tiny, dry patch on her cheek. She thought it was just one of those "age spots" or maybe a stubborn patch of dryness, but when it didn't go away, she finally saw a dermatologist. After some back-and-forth visits, a biopsy confirmed it was squamous cell carcinoma. Don't worry; this isn't as scary as it sounds—when caught early, it's one of the most treatable types of skin cancer. She went through a series of treatments, including surgery that took several hours, but thankfully, she's now cancer-free.

What Is Skin Cancer, and How Does It Sneak Up on Us?

Skin cancer often starts small—a rough patch, a red spot, or a sore that stubbornly refuses to heal. It's sneaky, sure, but it's not unstoppable. The good news? If caught early, it's more than 95% curable. But left unchecked, it can grow more comfortable than an uninvited houseguest—and none of us want that kind of "guest" on our face or body!

Certain factors put some people more at risk. If you have fair skin, light eyes, or a history of sunburns, you're in the higher-risk group. And if you love tanning beds, it's time to rethink that habit. While a bronzed glow might seem appealing, those intense UV rays are essentially fast-tracking your skin to damage—and, yes, potentially cancer. Here's a reality check: It's not just about beach days. Everyday moments, like gardening or driving, also expose your skin to cumulative UV damage over time.

Your Skin's Best Defense: Sunscreen and Smart Habits

The simplest and most effective way to protect your skin? Make sunscreen your ultimate sidekick. Look for a broad-spectrum sunscreen with at least SPF 30 (yes, there are lightweight, non-greasy options you'll actually enjoy using!) and apply it every morning. This isn't just for sunny days or outdoor adventures—even cloudy days and indoor lighting can expose your skin to harmful rays.

When heading out, top off your routine with a wide-brimmed hat and a pair of chic sunglasses. And as tempting as tanning beds might be, consider this your friendly nudge to skip them entirely. Trust me, your future self—and your skin—will thank you.

Do a Monthly Skin Check: It's Easier Than You Think

Think of a skin check as giving your body a little TLC. Every month or so, scan for any unusual spots: rough patches, scaly areas, or anything that doesn't seem to heal. This isn't about being paranoid; it's about being proactive. If something feels off or looks different, trust your gut and book an appointment with a dermatologist.

The Final Glow-Up: Protect and Preserve

The next time you're layering on your favorite serum or moisturizer, take an extra second to add some SPF into the mix. It's a small step that delivers big rewards—helping you maintain healthy, glowing skin for the long haul. Remember, the true glow comes from skin that's happy, healthy, and safe. So let's raise a (metaphorical) glass to smart sun care and keep our skin radiant for years to come!

CONCLUSION: EMBRACING HOLISTIC BEAUTY AND RADIANCE

At the core of holistic skincare lies a truth that resonates deeply: beauty isn't just skin deep—it's a reflection of the care and love you give to your entire self. Your skin is not merely a canvas to be polished; it's a vibrant storyteller of your health, your habits, and your lifestyle. This journey isn't about chasing perfection but embracing balance, self-compassion, and a commitment to nurturing your body, mind, and spirit.

Throughout this chapter, we've uncovered the powerful connection between your choices and your skin's health. From nourishing your body with nutrient-rich foods to protecting it from daily stressors, every action you take leaves its mark. And here's the empowering part: these choices are yours to make. You have the ability to transform your skin—and your life—one mindful step at a time.

There's no magic serum, no overnight fix that can promise life-long beauty. The true secret lies in cultivating habits that honor your body's needs, reflect your values, and align with your goals. Each time you care for your skin—whether through a thoughtful skincare routine, a balanced meal, or a moment of rest—you're making an investment in your health, confidence, and inner glow.

As you close this chapter, take a moment to reflect on what truly matters: not the fleeting pursuit of flawless skin, but the enduring strength and beauty that come from living intention-ally. Small, consistent actions—choosing better foods, priori-tizing self-care, and embracing healthy routines—have the power to create lasting change. Remember, the journey to radiant skin is a marathon, not a sprint. Each step, no matter how small, is a victory.

You deserve to look and feel radiant, confident, and strong. By committing to a holistic approach to skincare, you're not just enhancing your complexion—you're honoring the woman within. This isn't just about outer beauty; it's about celebrating the resilience, wisdom, and power that shine through when you prioritize yourself.

Let today be your beginning. Start with one choice, one step toward a more vibrant, healthier you. Watch as those choices blossom—on your skin, in your confidence, and in the life you build for yourself. You have the power, and you deserve nothing less than the beauty and strength that come from living fully, inside and out.

Here's to your journey—one choice, one step, one glow at a time.

CHAPTER 15

NATURAL REMEDIES FOR HAIR GROWTH AND BEAUTY

WHAT THEY DON'T TELL YOU ABOUT HAIR GROWTH—THE SECRET TO THICKER, STRONGER HAIR!

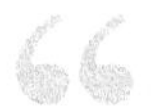 "Life is too short to have boring hair."

— Anonymous

Everyone wants long, luscious hair and thick, beautiful eyelashes. Although there are plenty of products on the market that claim to give you the results you desire, many of them are filled with harsh chemicals that can do more harm than good. Luckily, there are a few simple home remedies that can help you achieve the same goal without any negative side effects. In this chapter, we will discuss natural ways to grow your hair and boost your confidence.

I have always struggled with my hair. It has a naturally thin texture, and because of the stressors in my life, I've often dealt with hair loss. My eyelashes suffer from thinness as well. My daughter has been blessed with gorgeous, luscious hair, and whenever I brush it out for her, I think to myself, "I wish I could have this, too! You are so lucky, sweetheart!"

So, while combing her hair, I'd often joke with her by saying: "Can mommy have your hair? Will you sell it to mommy?" She would laugh and joke back: "Sure, I'll sell it to you for a million dollars mommy!". Although she's very young, she already understands the value of beautiful hair!

Through my attempts to improve my hair and eyelashes, I've turned to popular commercial hair treatments. I also got eyelash extensions. However, I noticed that by using these products and getting extensions, my hair suffered even more! It created a negative feedback loop where the products temporarily improved something, only to cause my hair to look worse, and I had to keep using the products to make it better for a short while. My natural eyelashes were falling out and looking worse than ever without extensions. These treatments simply did not give me the desired long-term results. So here's what I did: I returned to my cultural roots and sought out natural remedies that people have relied on for many generations to treat hair loss and thinning.

Let's look at some holistic ways to treat these issues.

EAT YOUR WAY TO BETTER HAIR AND EYELASHES

You probably know that eating a balanced diet is essential for overall health, but did you know it's just as important for the health of your hair and eyelashes? Yes, your diet directly impacts your hair's strength, growth, and shine. By making small, thoughtful changes to your meals, you can nourish your hair and even promote eyelash growth naturally.

Protein: The Foundation of Hair Health

Protein is the building block of strong, healthy hair. Your hair strands are made primarily of keratin, a type of protein, so it's no surprise that a protein deficiency can lead to weaker hair or even hair loss. When your body doesn't get enough protein, it prioritizes vital organs like your heart and brain, leaving little for non-essential areas like your hair follicles. This can leave your hair brittle, dry, and more prone to shedding.

To ensure your hair gets its fair share, include lean protein sources in every meal. Think chicken, fish, tofu, legumes, and eggs—these are all excellent choices to keep your hair looking and feeling strong.

Biotin: The Hair and Nail Superhero

Biotin, also known as Vitamin B7, is a water-soluble vitamin that's celebrated for its role in improving hair and nail health. Research suggests that biotin deficiency can lead to hair thinning, poor hair growth, and even brittle, dry strands.

You can find biotin naturally in foods like:

- Eggs
- Nuts and seeds (like almonds and sunflower seeds)
- Leafy green vegetables (like spinach and kale)
- Sweet potatoes

For those who might struggle to get enough biotin through food, a supplement can help. Just make sure not to exceed the recommended daily dose of 2.5 mg, as more isn't always better when it comes to vitamins.

A PERSONAL TOUCH: FUEL YOUR HAIR WITH LOVE

When I began incorporating more protein and biotin-rich foods into my meals, I noticed a significant improvement in my hair's texture and strength. My eyelashes, too, seemed fuller and healthier. It was like my hair had been waiting for the nutrients it needed to thrive!

Remember, every small choice adds up. When you feed your body the nutrients it craves, it rewards you with healthier hair, radiant skin, and more energy. So why not start today? Add a handful of nuts to your afternoon snack or swap out your usual side dish for a leafy green salad. Your hair—and lashes—will thank you for the extra care.

THE POWER OF OMEGA-3 FATTY ACIDS FOR SCALP HEALTH AND HAIR GROWTH

Did you know that your scalp plays a vital role in determining the health of your hair? A nourished, inflammation-free scalp is the foundation for strong, beautiful strands. This is where omega-3 fatty acids come in, acting as a superhero for your scalp and hair health. These healthy fats are not only great for your heart and brain, but they're also essential for maintaining a hydrated scalp, reducing inflammation, and promoting hair growth.

Why Omega-3 Fatty Acids Matter

Omega-3 fatty acids are essential fats that your body can't produce on its own, so you need to get them from your diet or supplements. They:

- **Moisturize Your Scalp:** Omega-3s help regulate your scalp's natural oil production, preventing dryness and flakiness.
- **Strengthen Hair Follicles:** These fats nourish the hair follicles, improving hair strength and reducing breakage.
- **Reduce Inflammation:** One of the most significant benefits is their ability to combat inflammation in the scalp, which can contribute to hair loss.

Why Does Scalp Inflammation Lead to Hair Loss?

Inflammation occurs when your body's immune system goes into overdrive, often in response to stress, infections, or nutrient imbalances. While inflammation is a natural defense mechanism, chronic inflammation in the scalp can be harmful.

Here's how it works:

1. **Hair Follicles Under Attack:** When inflammation takes over, your immune system may mistakenly target your hair follicles, treating them like foreign invaders. This immune response can damage the follicles, causing them to shrink and eventually stop producing hair altogether—a condition known as alopecia areata.
2. **Nutrient Blockage:** Inflammation can also restrict blood flow to the scalp, cutting off the delivery of essential nutrients and oxygen to the hair roots. Without these nutrients, the follicles weaken, and hair growth slows down.
3. **Damaged Scalp Environment:** A chronically inflamed scalp becomes an unhealthy environment for hair growth, leading to thinning, shedding, and even permanent hair loss if left untreated.

How Omega-3s Help Combat Scalp Inflammation

Omega-3 fatty acids are anti-inflammatory powerhouses. They help regulate the production of inflammatory molecules in the body, reducing swelling and irritation in the scalp. By calming the immune response, omega-3s create a healthier environment for your hair follicles to thrive.

- **Promotes Scalp Hydration:** Omega-3s help retain moisture in the scalp, preventing the dryness and itchiness that can often accompany inflammation.
- **Strengthens Follicle Function:** By improving the overall health of the scalp, omega-3s support stronger, healthier hair growth.

Sources of Omega-3 Fatty Acids

Getting your dose of omega-3s is easier than you think! Here are some excellent sources to incorporate into your diet:

- **Fatty Fish:** Salmon, mackerel, sardines, and herring are rich in omega-3s and packed with other nutrients like protein and vitamin D, both of which are essential for hair growth.

- **Plant-Based Options:** Flaxseeds, chia seeds, walnuts, and hemp seeds are great alternatives if you're not a fan of fish or follow a plant-based diet.
- **Supplements:** If dietary sources aren't enough, omega-3 supplements like fish oil or algae-based omega-3 capsules can be a convenient way to ensure you're getting the right amount.

A PERSONAL NOTE

Let me share a little story with you. I used to wonder why my scalp felt so dry and itchy during stressful weeks. And the shedding? Let's just say it wasn't pretty. That's when I discovered omega-3s and their magic. After a few months of incorporating more salmon and chia seeds into my meals, my scalp felt less irritated, and my hair loss noticeably reduced. It was a game-changer!

So, if you're struggling with hair thinning or scalp issues, start with your plate. Adding omega-3-rich foods to your diet is a simple yet effective way to support your scalp and hair health. Your hair deserves all the love, and it starts with nourishing your scalp from the inside out.

You can get omega-3s from fatty fish such as salmon, mackerel, and herring, or from plant-based sources such as flaxseeds and chia seeds.

If you're looking for ways to improve the health of your hair and eyelashes, look no further than your kitchen! By including some key nutrients in your diet, you can promote hair growth and prevent hair loss. So stock up on protein-rich foods like chicken and fish, load up on leafy greens for biotin, and add some omega-3-rich foods like salmon or flaxseeds to your meals —your hair (and eyelashes) will thank you!

Because of my hair-thinning experience, I have carried out extensive research on the best types of food to eat and which natural hair treatment options work best to prevent or reduce hair loss. This is what I am sharing with you in this chapter, as I have seen amazing results with my hair and skin. They are also great for other body parts, so it's a win-win scenario.

THE SCIENCE BEHIND NATURAL INGREDIENTS FOR HAIR GROWTH

Understanding the science behind these natural remedies not only makes them more credible but also helps you appreciate why they work. Let's dive into the research and explore how these ingredients boost hair growth.

Apple Cider Vinegar (ACV): Balancing the Scalp's pH

Your scalp has a natural pH level of around 5.5, which is slightly acidic. Many hair products, however, can disrupt this balance, making the scalp more alkaline and prone to dandruff, dryness, and fungal growth. The acidic nature of ACV restores the scalp's pH, creating an environment that discourages harmful microbes.

How It Promotes Hair Growth:

- **Exfoliation:** ACV gently removes dead skin cells and buildup that clog hair follicles, allowing hair to grow unimpeded.
- **Improved Circulation:** By cleaning the scalp, ACV boosts blood flow to the hair follicles, delivering essential nutrients.
- **Antimicrobial Properties:** It contains acetic acid, which fights bacteria and fungi that can weaken the hair shaft and cause shedding.

Coconut Oil: Deep Nourishment for Scalp and Hair

Coconut oil is rich in medium-chain fatty acids, particularly lauric acid, which penetrates the hair shaft more effectively than other oils. This helps strengthen the hair from within and prevents protein loss.

How It Promotes Hair Growth:

- **Moisturization:** Coconut oil locks in moisture, preventing dryness that can lead to breakage.
- **Anti-Microbial Action:** Lauric acid inhibits the growth of harmful bacteria and fungi on the scalp, reducing dandruff and irritation.
- **Reduced Protein Loss:** By sealing the cuticle, coconut oil protects hair proteins that are essential for strength and elasticity.

Aloe Vera: The Cooling Healer

Aloe vera contains enzymes, like proteolytic enzymes, that repair dead skin cells on the scalp. This not only promotes hair growth but also keeps the scalp hydrated and itch-free.

How It Promotes Hair Growth:

- **Anti-Inflammatory Properties:** Aloe vera reduces inflammation, a common cause of hair loss.
- **Hydration:** Its gel-like consistency provides deep moisturization without making the scalp greasy.
- **Rich in Nutrients:** Aloe vera contains vitamins A, C, and E, which help regenerate new hair cells and strengthen existing ones.

Fenugreek Seeds: Nature's Hormone Booster

Fenugreek seeds are rich in phytoestrogens (plant-based compounds that mimic estrogen), which can help balance hormonal imbalances that lead to hair thinning. They also contain nicotinic acid (a form of vitamin B3) and lecithin, which nourish hair follicles.

How It Promotes Hair Growth:

- **Hormonal Support:** The phytoestrogens stimulate hair growth in cases of hormone-related hair loss.
- **Anti-Inflammatory Action:** Fenugreek reduces scalp inflammation, ensuring a healthier environment for hair growth.
- **Strength and Shine:** Its rich lecithin content coats the hair, adding shine and strength while preventing breakage.

Rice Water: Nutrient-Rich Elixir

Rice water contains inositol, a carbohydrate that penetrates the hair shaft to repair damage and improve elasticity. Additionally, its amino acids and vitamins nourish the scalp and hair follicles.

How It Promotes Hair Growth:

- **Repair and Strength:** Inositol strengthens hair from the root, reducing breakage.
- **Improved Elasticity:** By coating the hair shaft, rice water improves its flexibility, preventing it from snapping.
- **Anti-Aging Benefits:** Rice water's antioxidants combat oxidative stress, which can prematurely age the scalp and weaken hair.

FINAL THOUGHTS ON THE SCIENCE OF HAIR CARE

Each of these ingredients is backed by science, demonstrating its potential to nourish the scalp, strengthen hair, and promote growth. By incorporating these natural remedies into your routine, you're not only caring for your hair but also supporting a healthier scalp environment—because healthy hair starts at the root!

Remember, consistency is the secret ingredient. Whether it's a weekly fenugreek paste or a quick rinse with rice water, these small habits can lead to big transformations over time. Your hair deserves this TLC, and the results will be worth it.

HOW TO KEEP HEALTHY EYELASHES

We all want longer, luscious lashes. Fortunately, there are a few things you can do to achieve this without resorting to harsh chemicals or fake lashes.

Nowadays, there are so many fake eyelashes sold on the market, and we, as women, all agree how convenient it is to use fake eyelashes to enhance beauty. While using these fake eyelashes, have you considered the potential harmful effects of the eyelash glue? It is pretty astonishing to note that lash glue is one of the most harmful beauty products on the market, with many of them containing toxic chemicals like ammonia, lead, and formaldehyde. These chemicals can damage your skin—causing complications like redness and inflammation. You should definitely be careful about using these products!

Here are a few of my favorite tips for growing longer eyelashes naturally.

1. **Castor oil** is one of the most popular natural remedies for hair growth, and that includes eyelashes. The fatty acids in castor oil help to nourish and condition your lashes, making them stronger and less likely to fall out. Just apply a small amount of castor oil to a clean mascara brush and brush it through your lashes before bedtime. I view castor oil as a truly impressive resource, as you can use it for both your hair and eyelashes. Yes, it's quite wonderful! However, like other discussed products, the key is consistent usage and patience while you wait to get the results you want.

2. **Green tea:** It sounds weird to consider green tea for your hair and eyelashes, but surprisingly, it provides

amazing benefits! Now, you might roll your eyes and say "really, green tea can help with hair and eyelashes? Yes, one stone can kill two birds. By sipping warm, fresh green tea, you're providing your body with an excellent amount of antioxidants to help your hair and eyelashes at the same time. So, after you finish drinking green tea, don't waste or throw away the rest. You can utilize the tea bag and the leftover tea for your eyelashes and hair! Not only is green tea full of antioxidants, but it also contains EGCG (which stands for epigallocatechin gallate). This substance can prevent hair loss by stopping the activity of hormones that cause hair loss. At the same time, it can nourish and stimulate the hair follicles to promote hair growth. Just brew a cup of green tea and allow it to cool. Once it's cooled, soak a clean cotton ball in the tea and apply it to your eyelashes. Leave it on for 5-10 minutes, then rinse with warm water.

3. **Coconut oil**, yes, I mentioned again! When applying it to your hair, don't forget to apply it to your eyelashes as well. It is truly another great option for growing longer eyelashes naturally. The nutrients in coconut oil help to strengthen hair follicles and promote growth. Just apply a small amount of coconut oil to a clean mascara brush and brush it through your lashes before bedtime.

ACTIONABLE TIPS FOR THINNING HAIR: CHOOSING THE RIGHT SHAMPOO AND UNDERSTANDING WATER'S ROLE

Thinning hair can feel like a challenge, but with the right knowledge and approach, you can help your hair thrive. Let's break down some science-backed and practical tips to empower you to make the best choices for your hair—and yes, we're even talking about water because it matters more than you might think!

Choosing the Right Shampoo for Thinning Hair

Your shampoo isn't just about cleaning your hair—it's the foundation of your hair care routine. Here's how to choose wisely:

1. **Go for Lightweight Formulas**
   - Why it matters: Thick, creamy shampoos can weigh your hair down, leaving it flat and lifeless.
   - What to look for: Clear shampoos are often less heavy and more suitable for fine or thinning hair.
2. **Seek Out Strengthening Ingredients**
   - Biotin: Known for promoting keratin production, biotin helps strengthen hair and reduce breakage.
   - Panthenol: A form of Vitamin B5, panthenol helps improve hair's elasticity and moisture retention.
   - Keratin: This protein fortifies the hair shaft, making it less prone to breakage.
3. **Avoid Harsh Chemicals**
   - Skip sulfates and parabens—they strip your hair of its natural oils and can exacerbate dryness and breakage.
   - Watch out for "fragrance" or "parfum" on the ingredient list, which often indicates hidden chemicals that can irritate sensitive scalps.
4. **Scalp Care is Key**
   - Look for shampoos with tea tree oil, aloe vera, or salicylic acid to gently cleanse and soothe your scalp, reducing inflammation that can lead to hair loss.

Does Water Type Impact Hair?

Yes, the type of water you wash your hair with can significantly affect its health. Let's dive into the details:

1. **Soft Water vs. Hard Water**
   - Soft Water: Gentle on your hair, it allows shampoos to lather more easily and prevents

buildup. Soft water helps keep your hair feeling soft and manageable.

- Hard Water: Contains high levels of minerals like calcium and magnesium, which can leave residue on your scalp and hair, causing it to feel dry and brittle. Over time, this buildup can lead to dullness and breakage.

2. **Pro Tip:** If you live in a hard water area, investing in a shower filter can make a world of difference. Filters help remove excess minerals, giving your hair a fighting chance to stay healthy.

3. **Filtered Water vs. Alkaline Water**
   - Filtered Water: Removes impurities, chlorine, and heavy metals that can irritate the scalp and damage hair.
   - Alkaline Water: While there's limited scientific evidence specifically linking alkaline water to hair health, its higher pH can help balance an overly acidic scalp, promoting a healthier environment for hair growth.

4. **Verdict:** If you're experiencing persistent scalp issues or hair loss, consider investing in a water filter for your shower. It's a simple yet effective way to improve the quality of the water you're using.

FINAL THOUGHTS ON WATER AND SHAMPOO FOR THINNING HAIR

Hair thinning can feel overwhelming, but it's manageable with the right care. Start by choosing a shampoo tailored to your hair's needs—one with strengthening ingredients and free of harsh chemicals. Pay attention to your water quality, as hard water can be a hidden culprit in hair damage. A water filter is a worthwhile investment, especially if you live in a hard water area.

Remember, hair care is a journey, not a race. Small, consistent changes—like choosing the right shampoo and being mindful of your water—can lead to big improvements over time. You're not just taking care of your hair; you're reclaiming your confidence and showing yourself some well-deserved love. Let's raise a glass of filtered water to that! 🥂

CHAPTER 16
AGING GRACEFULLY
A HOLISTIC GUIDE TO RADIANCE AND RESILIENCE

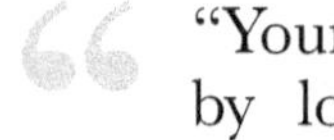

"Your face is marked with lines of life, put there by love and laughter, suffering and tears. It's beautiful."

— Lynsay Sands

THE ART AND JOY OF AGING GRACEFULLY

Let's face it—aging isn't a problem to be solved but a journey to be embraced. Those fine lines? They're the marks of wisdom, laughter, and a life well-lived. As someone who's weathered the sleepless nights of motherhood, the stresses of work, and the occasional shock of seeing a new wrinkle in the mirror, I understand. Aging brings change, yes, but it also brings opportunity—the chance to care for ourselves in deeper, more meaningful ways.

As I've shared in previous chapters, we've explored how to minimize fine lines and reduce wrinkles. And yes, we do our best with the tools we have. But let's take a moment to reframe how we see those lines when they inevitably appear. Don't beat yourself up over them. Instead, think of them as your personal map—etched with stories of love, resilience, and growth. We can't stop the aging process entirely, but we can slow it down and, more importantly, celebrate every milestone along the way.

Aging gracefully isn't about chasing perfection; it's about finding joy and beauty in the here and now. Together, we'll dive into ways to nurture your body, mind, and spirit—blending timeless wisdom with modern science. From the foods that fuel your glow to the mindset shifts that spark your confidence, this is your guide to feeling radiant and resilient.

Because every stage of life brings its own kind of beauty. Every laugh line is a reminder of the moments that made you smile. Every milestone is a chapter in your incredible story. Aging gracefully isn't a battle—it's an honor. So let's celebrate it together, embracing the journey with open arms and a whole lot of love for ourselves.

Here's an expanded version of the holistic approaches for aging gracefully, tailored for women, with a conversational and friendly tone. Light humor is sprinkled in to keep it engaging without diminishing the importance of the subject.

MINDSET AND MENTAL RESILIENCE: AGING STARTS FROM WITHIN

Ladies, let's start with the truth bomb: aging gracefully isn't just about wrinkle creams or serums. It starts in your head—yep, right up there. A positive mindset can do wonders for your overall well-being. Think of it as the anti-aging elixir your soul craves (and it's free!).

- **Gratitude Is Your Superpower:** Studies have shown that practicing gratitude can reduce stress, boost happiness, and even improve your immune system. Start a gratitude journal and jot down three things you're thankful for every day. "My coffee didn't spill this morning" totally counts!
- **Stay Socially Connected:** Don't let age be an excuse to retreat into isolation. Call that friend you've

been meaning to catch up with, join a book club, or even try a dance class. Connections keep your brain sharp and your heart happy.

- **Learn Something New:** Lifelong learning isn't just for the young. Whether it's mastering sourdough bread (finally) or learning Italian for that dream vacation, keeping your brain active boosts confidence and keeps you curious. Plus, nothing feels more empowering than nailing a new skill and casually mentioning it over brunch.

HORMONAL HEALTH: NAVIGATING THE SHIFTS WITH GRACE

Ah, hormones—the drama queens of our bodies. As we age, they like to shake things up, leading to mood swings, energy dips, and changes in skin and hair. But don't worry; there are ways to keep these divas in check.

- **Support With Phytoestrogens:** Foods like soy, flaxseeds, and chickpeas contain plant-based estrogens that can help balance hormones naturally. Add them to your diet for a little hormonal harmony.
- **Adaptogenic Herbs:** Ever heard of ashwagandha or maca root? These herbs are like your hormonal cheerleaders, helping your body adapt to stress and maintain balance. Consider adding them to smoothies or teas—but check with your doctor first, just to be safe.
- **Exercise for Balance:** A little yoga or Pilates can do wonders for hormonal health. These gentle movements help regulate cortisol (that pesky stress hormone) and keep you feeling centered. Plus, who doesn't love an excuse to buy cute yoga pants?

FUNCTIONAL FITNESS AND POSTURE: STANDING TALL, AGING STRONG

Let's talk posture, ladies. Slouching isn't just bad for your back —it's also not doing you any favors in the confidence department. The good news? Functional fitness can help you stay strong, upright, and fabulous.

- **Strength Training:** Lifting light weights or using resistance bands is a game-changer. Not only does it improve muscle tone, but it also supports bone density, which we all know becomes crucial as we age. Bonus: carrying groceries feels like less of a workout!
- **Balance and Core Work:** Exercises like planks, lunges, or even standing on one leg while brushing your teeth (yes, try it!) can improve balance and prevent falls. After all, we're aiming for graceful, not wobbly.
- **Stretch It Out:** A few simple stretches every morning can improve flexibility and reduce stiffness. Picture yourself as a cat stretching after a nap—relaxed yet ready to conquer the day.

COGNITIVE HEALTH: KEEP THAT BRAIN BUZZING

A sharp mind is one of the greatest gifts of aging gracefully. And no, you don't have to dive into quantum physics to keep your brain sharp (unless that's your thing—then go for it!).

- **Brain-Boosting Foods:** Load up on omega-3-rich foods like salmon, walnuts, and chia seeds. These are brain food, literally. Your neurons will thank you.
- **Mental Workouts:** Crossword puzzles, Sudoku, or even a good mystery novel can keep your brain engaged. Think of it as a workout for your mind—no gym membership required.

- **Mindfulness and Meditation:** Sometimes, the best thing you can do for your brain is nothing. Meditation reduces stress, enhances focus, and helps you embrace the present moment. Start with just five minutes a day. Theres no need to contort yourself into a pretzel—just sit, breathe, and let go.

CREATIVE AGING: REDISCOVERING JOY AND PURPOSE

Who says aging means slowing down? This is the perfect time to dive into something new or rekindle an old passion. Think of it as your golden ticket to self-expression.

- **Try a New Hobby:** Whether it's painting, gardening, or baking artisan bread (hello, Instagram-worthy loaves), hobbies keep your mind engaged and your heart fulfilled. They're also a great way to meet like-minded people.
- **Share Your Wisdom:** Mentor someone in your field or start a blog about your journey. Your experience is a treasure trove for others, and sharing it can be deeply rewarding.
- **Travel (Even Locally):** You don't have to jet off to Paris to explore. A nearby town or a scenic hike can bring new perspectives and adventures.

AGING GRACEFULLY: IT'S ALL ABOUT BALANCE

At its core, aging gracefully is about finding balance—nurturing your body, feeding your mind, and fueling your soul. It's about embracing the changes, celebrating the milestones, and showing up for yourself every day. Remember, this is your time to shine. You've earned every laugh line, every strand of wisdom (gray hair counts!), and every ounce of joy you bring to the world.

Let's make aging not just graceful but downright fabulous. Because you're not just aging—you're thriving. Let's toast to that—green smoothie or wine glass, your call!

SECTION 1: THE POWER TRIO OF SKIN HEALTH – COLLAGEN, ELASTIN, AND HYALURONIC ACID

Now that we've talked about the importance of mindset, resilience, and holistic health, let's dive into some skin-loving essentials. Aging gracefully doesn't mean we can't give our skin the best tools to thrive. And when it comes to keeping your skin firm, elastic, and glowing, three key players take the stage: **collagen**, **elastin**, and **hyaluronic acid**.

These superstars are like the building blocks of youthful skin. Think of collagen as the foundation, elastin as the springy trampoline, and hyaluronic acid as the ultimate hydration wizard. Here's how to support them naturally—because your skin deserves a little love!

Collagen: The Skin's Firm Foundation

Collagen is what gives your skin that firm, smooth texture we all admire. It's like scaffolding for your skin, but as we age, collagen production slows down, leading to sagging and fine lines. Supporting collagen doesn't mean chasing expensive creams—it's easier (and tastier!) than you think.

- **How to Boost It Naturally:** One word: broth. If you've ever savored a comforting bowl of Vietnamese "pho," you've already given your skin a collagen treat. Bone broth made from beef or chicken bones is a natural source of collagen. Add in some tendons or even a splash of fish sauce (another collagen-rich ingredient), and you're treating your skin from the inside out. Bonus: it's delicious!

- **Pro-Tip:** Don't love broth? Try collagen supplements, but check the label for clean, high-quality sources.

Elastin: The Skin's "Bounce-Back" Factor

Remember when your skin could spring back into place without a care in the world? That's elastin at work. As we age, elastin production slows, which can make skin less resilient. But don't worry—this is where Mother Nature comes to the rescue.

- **How to Help Elastin Thrive:** Stock up on vitamin C-rich foods like strawberries, bell peppers, and oranges. Vitamin C isn't just a cold-fighter—it's a critical player in the production of elastin. And don't forget dark leafy greens like spinach and kale. These nutritional powerhouses give your skin the bounce it needs.
- **Easy Tip:** Add some sliced bell peppers to your salads or blend spinach into a smoothie. It's a quick, tasty way to help your skin snap back with ease.

Hyaluronic Acid: The Ultimate Moisture Magnet

Hyaluronic acid is the MVP of hydration. This magical molecule holds up to 1,000 times its weight in water, making it a must-have for keeping skin plump, dewy, and youthful. While topical serums are great, feeding your skin from within is just as effective.

- **Nourish It Naturally:** Foods like spinach, nuts, seeds, and soy are rich in the amino acids and magnesium needed for hyaluronic acid production. Sprinkle some chia seeds on your yogurt or snack on almonds to keep your skin hydrated from the inside out.
- **Quick Hydration Hack:** Stay hydrated by sipping water throughout the day, but make it fun! Add a slice of cucumber or a squeeze of lemon for an

antioxidant boost alongside your hyaluronic acid-rich diet.

By understanding and supporting these three powerhouses—collagen, elastin, and hyaluronic acid—you're giving your skin the foundation it needs to age gracefully. Think of each bite of nutrient-packed food as a little love note to your future self. Aging is inevitable, but thriving while we do it? That's the goal—and with this trio on your side, it's absolutely possible.

SECTION 2: ANTIOXIDANTS – YOUR SKIN'S BEST DEFENSE AGAINST AGING

Antioxidants are the unsung heroes in the fight against aging, protecting skin cells from free radical damage. Free radicals are the pesky molecules that damage skin's structure, leading to dullness and wrinkles. Here's how to get your daily dose of antioxidants—and maybe even make grocery shopping a little more exciting!

Smart Antioxidant Choices for Everyday

You don't need fancy or expensive foods to reap the benefits of antioxidants. Blueberries, spinach, and tomatoes are all packed with antioxidants and are budget-friendly, too. Add them to your weekly grocery list and keep it simple.

- **Cooked vs. Raw:** When it comes to maximizing antioxidants, how you prepare foods can make a difference. Tomatoes, for instance, release more lycopene (a powerful antioxidant) when cooked. But foods like berries and spinach retain more nutrients in their raw form. Aim for a mix of cooked and raw to get the best of both worlds!
- **Color-Coding Your Cart:** When shopping, look for color-rich produce, like red, blue, orange, and green fruits and vegetables. These colors typically indicate antioxidant-rich foods. A "rainbow plate" isn't just a

trend—it's a skin-nourishing strategy that keeps your meals vibrant and nutrient-dense.

SECTION 3: HYDRATION HACKS FOR SUPPLE, GLOWING SKIN

Hydration is one of the simplest yet most powerful tools in your skin's anti-aging arsenal. It's essential for a healthy complexion, promoting elasticity and helping skin stay smooth and radiant. While foods like cucumber and watermelon offer a nice hydration boost, maintaining a steady intake of water throughout the day is key.

Daily Water Reminders for Skin Health

Let's be real: remembering to drink enough water can be a challenge, especially with busy schedules. One easy hack is to keep a 2-liter bottle on your desk or within sight as a visual reminder. Treat it as your daily hydration goal—finish the bottle by the end of the day, and you're set!

Spice Up Your Sips

Plain water isn't the only option for hydration. Herbal teas and infused waters can make hydration more enjoyable. Try adding cucumber, lemon, or mint for a refreshing twist that not only boosts hydration but also provides extra antioxidants. So if you find plain water too bland, give these a try to keep things interesting and your skin glowing.

By focusing on these essentials—collagen, elastin, hyaluronic acid, antioxidants, and hydration—you're giving your skin the very best support for graceful aging. Each choice you make, from sipping broth to savoring berries, is a step toward glowing skin that reflects the vitality and joy of every season of life.

ANTIOXIDANTS, HYDRATION, AND HEALTHY FATS: THE GLOW-UP TRIO FOR EVERY STAGE OF LIFE

Aging isn't about losing your glow; it's about finding new ways to shine. Antioxidants, hydration, and healthy fats are like your dream team—working behind the scenes to keep your skin radiant, your mind sharp, and your energy unstoppable. Let's dive into how these superstar nutrients can help you age gracefully while feeling absolutely fabulous.

Antioxidants: Your Skin's Invisible Shield

Think of antioxidants as your personal bodyguards against life's stressors. They fight off free radicals—those pesky troublemakers responsible for wrinkles, dull skin, and that "Why do I look so tired?" feeling. But antioxidants aren't just about appearances; they protect your heart, brain, and overall vitality, too.

Why Antioxidants Are a Must-Have:

- **Cellular Repair Magic:** Antioxidants help your skin bounce back from daily stressors like pollution, sun exposure, and late nights.
- **Collagen's Best Friend:** Vitamin C and beta-carotene team up to keep your skin plump and elastic.
- **Brain Boosters:** Flavonoids and polyphenols support mental clarity—because who doesn't want a sharp mind to match their glowing skin?

Your Antioxidant Playbook:

- **Snack on Blueberries:** These little gems pack a powerful punch. Toss them in your oatmeal or eat them by the handful—your skin will thank you.
- **Sip Golden Turmeric Tea:** Turmeric isn't just a trend; its curcumin content fights inflammation like a

pro. Add a sprinkle to soups or try a warm turmeric latte for an anti-aging boost.

- **Roast Those Tomatoes:** Cooked tomatoes release lycopene, a skin-protecting powerhouse. Serve them in soups, sauces, or as a side dish, and let your skin soak up the benefits.

Hydration: The Real Fountain of Youth

We've all heard it: "Drink more water!" But let's be honest—it's easier said than done. As we age, our skin gets drier, and staying hydrated becomes non-negotiable. Hydration isn't just about quenching your thirst; it's about keeping your skin dewy, your energy up, and your body running like a well-oiled machine.

Hydration Hacks to Make It Fun:

- **Make Water Irresistible:** Add slices of cucumber, lemon, or mint to your water for a spa-like experience. Bored with plain water? Try sparkling water with a splash of fruit juice for a bubbly treat.
- **Hydrating Snacks:** Keep cucumber slices, watermelon chunks, and celery sticks on hand. These hydrating heroes double as tasty, guilt-free snacks.
- **Track It Stylishly:** Get a cute water bottle with time markers. It's like having a hydration coach cheering you on all day long.

Pro Tip: If you love coffee (don't we all?), balance it out with an extra glass of water. Caffeine can dehydrate you, but a little extra H2O keeps things in check.

Healthy Fats: Glow-Up from the Inside Out

Whoever said "fat is bad" clearly never met avocados or walnuts. Healthy fats are your secret weapon for soft, supple skin, shiny hair, and even a sharper mind. They're like the beauty elixir you didn't know you needed.

Why Healthy Fats Are Your Skin's BFF:

- **Skin Hydration Savior:** Omega-3 fatty acids lock in moisture, keeping your skin from looking dry or flaky.
- **Inflammation Fighter:** Healthy fats calm inflammation, reducing redness and irritation.
- **Brain Fuel:** DHA, a type of omega-3, supports memory and focus—because you're aging gracefully, not forgetfully!

How to Add Them Without Overthinking:

- **Avocado Love:** Spread it on toast, toss it in a salad, or blend it into a smoothie. It's creamy, dreamy, and oh-so-good for your skin.
- **Nutty Snacks:** A handful of walnuts or almonds is all it takes to add a glow-boosting dose of omega-3s.
- **Seed Sprinkles:** Chia and flaxseeds are tiny but mighty. Add them to yogurt, oatmeal, or even baked goods for a nutrient-packed kick.

Why This Trio Matters for Women

Antioxidants, hydration, and healthy fats aren't just about looking good—they're about feeling empowered, vibrant, and strong at every age. These aren't quick fixes or fads; they're sustainable habits that celebrate your body's resilience and beauty.

Empowering Takeaway: You don't need expensive creams or complicated routines to age gracefully. You just need a handful of blueberries, a refreshing glass of water, and a sprinkle of seeds. Small, intentional choices add up to big results. So, start today—your glow-up journey begins now.

SECTION 4: EXERCISE AND STRENGTH TRAINING FOR A YOUTHFUL BODY

Let's face it, we can't turn back time, but we can definitely outsmart it with a little movement. Staying active isn't just about keeping fit; it's your secret weapon to feeling fabulous at any age. Whether it's lifting weights to build strength or stretching those laugh lines with facial yoga, exercise helps you stay strong, energized, and confident. The best part? These practices are simple, enjoyable, and can easily become a natural part of your weekly routine. With just a little effort, you can glow from head to toe and embrace every year with vitality and grace.

Strength Training: Build Strength for a Resilient Body

Strength training isn't about bulking up—it's about maintaining muscle tone, supporting a healthy metabolism, and keeping bones strong as you age. And the best part? It doesn't take hours in the gym to see results.

- **Exercises to Try:** Squats, lunges, and light resistance exercises are perfect for keeping muscles toned and strong. Aim to do these exercises two to three times a week. Resistance bands or light weights are great tools to enhance these moves.
- **The Benefits:** By strengthening muscles, you're supporting your joints, improving balance, and even boosting your metabolism, which tends to slow with age. This kind of exercise makes day-to-day tasks easier, and your body feels more resilient and youthful.

Strength training for just a few minutes a day, a couple of times a week, can help you feel capable and confident at any age.

Facial Yoga: Your Secret to a Toned, Youthful Face

While you're strengthening your body, don't forget your face! Facial yoga is a natural, non-invasive way to lift, tone, and firm your face. This simple routine only takes a few minutes a day, but it can make a big difference in reducing tension, promoting circulation, and enhancing your skin's firmness.

Here's a simple facial yoga routine to add to your daily beauty ritual:

1. Cheek Lifts

- **Purpose:** Tones cheeks, reduces sagging, and promotes circulation.
- **Steps:** Sit comfortably, shoulders relaxed. Form a gentle smile, lifting the corners of your mouth slightly. Press down gently on each cheek with your fingers, and lift your cheeks toward your eyes against this gentle resistance. Hold for 5 seconds, then release. Repeat 10 times.

2. Jawline Definer

- **Purpose:** Strengthens the jawline, reduces the double chin, and defines contours.
- **Steps:** Tilt your head back slightly and look up. Press your tongue to the roof of your mouth, then move your lower lip over your upper lip as far as possible. Hold for 5 seconds, feeling the stretch along your jawline. Return to a neutral position and relax. Repeat 10 times.

3. Forehead Smoother (Brow Lift)

- **Purpose:** Reduces forehead lines and lifts the brows for a refreshed look.
- **Steps:** Place your fingers just above each eyebrow. Gently press down as you try to raise your eyebrows.

Hold for 5 seconds, feeling the resistance, then relax. Repeat this movement 10 times.

4. Eye Brightener

- **Purpose:** Lifts and tones the area around the eyes, reducing puffiness and dark circles.
- **Steps:** Form a "V" shape with your index and middle fingers around each eye, placing one finger on the inner corner and one on the outer. Gently press down as you squint your lower eyelids upward (you should feel a slight pull under your eyes). Hold for 3 seconds, then relax. Repeat 10 times.

5. Smile Line Eraser

- **Purpose:** Softens smile lines and boosts cheek firmness.
- **Steps:** Place your fingertips on the apples of your cheeks and press down slightly as you smile. Hold the smile for 5 seconds, feeling the tension in your cheeks, then release. Repeat 10 times.

This entire face yoga routine takes just 5–10 minutes, but practicing it consistently can refresh your facial features, reduce tension, and even lift your mood. With each repetition, you're strengthening muscles that will help your face stay firm and youthful. And the best part? These exercises can be done anywhere—no equipment or gym membership is required.

Strength Training: Build Strength for a Resilient Body

Strength training isn't about bulking up or competing with gym buffs—it's about celebrating and preserving the strength that carries you through life. As we age, muscle tone naturally declines, but with just a few simple exercises, you can reclaim that strength, support a healthy metabolism, and keep your bones as sturdy as ever. The best part? You don't need hours at the gym to see results—this is about working smarter, not harder.

Why Strength Training Matters

Strength training keeps your body strong, your posture upright, and your joints supported. It also revs up your metabolism, which tends to slow down with age, and boosts your balance, making everyday tasks easier and reducing the risk of injuries.

Try These Simple Moves

- **Squats and Lunges:** Strengthen your legs and core with these classics. Start without weights and add resistance bands or light dumbbells when you're ready for a challenge.
- **Arm Raises and Push-Ups:** Keep your upper body toned and strong. Modify push-ups by doing them on your knees or against a wall if needed.
- **Plank Variations:** Tone your core and improve your balance. Start with a basic plank and work up to side planks for extra oblique strength.

Pro Tip: Commit to just 15–20 minutes twice a week. That's all it takes to feel stronger, more capable, and confident at any age.

Facial Yoga: Your Secret to a Youthful Glow

Now that your body is getting its workout, let's talk about your face. Yes, your face has muscles too, and they deserve some love! Facial yoga is a natural, non-invasive way to lift, tone, and firm your face, leaving you looking refreshed and radiant. It's quick, easy, and might even make you giggle while you're doing it (bonus points for boosting your mood!).

Why Facial Yoga?

- It improves circulation, bringing a healthy glow to your skin.
- It tones facial muscles, reducing the appearance of sagging and wrinkles.
- It's a great way to relieve tension—goodbye, clenched jaw and furrowed brows!

Your Go-To Facial Yoga Routine

1. **Cheek Lifts:**
   - What It Does: Lifts and tones sagging cheeks.
   - How to Do It: Smile gently and press your fingers onto your cheeks. Lift your cheeks toward your eyes against the light pressure. Hold for 5 seconds, then release. Repeat 10 times.
2. **Jawline Definer:**
   - What It Does: Tightens the jawline and reduces double chin.
   - How to Do It: Tilt your head back slightly, press your tongue to the roof of your mouth, and stretch your lower lip over your upper lip. Hold for 5 seconds, relax, and repeat 10 times.
3. **Forehead Smoother:**
   - What It Does: Softens forehead lines and lifts brows.
   - How to Do It: Place your fingers just above your brows, press lightly, and try to lift your eyebrows. Feel the resistance, hold for 5 seconds, and relax. Repeat 10 times.
4. **Eye Brightener:**
   - What It Does: Reduces puffiness and tones the delicate eye area.
   - How to Do It: Create a "V" shape with your fingers, placing them at the inner and outer corners of your eyes. Gently press down as you

squint your lower eyelids upward. Hold for 3 seconds and relax. Repeat 10 times.

5. **Smile Line Eraser:**
   - What It Does: Softens smile lines and boosts cheek firmness.
   - How to Do It: Smile and press your fingertips on the apples of your cheeks. Hold the smile for 5 seconds and release. Repeat 10 times.

Pulling It All Together

By weaving strength training and facial yoga into your weekly routine, you're not just investing in your health—you're celebrating the beauty of your body at every stage of life. Strength training tones your muscles and keeps you agile, while facial yoga keeps your glow intact and your features lifted.

Aging Gracefully in Action: Aging isn't about holding on to the past; it's about embracing your present with strength and grace. So, grab those weights, stretch those cheeks, and feel the joy of movement as you age vibrantly. With just a little effort and a lot of self-love, you're building resilience, confidence, and beauty from the inside out.

Remember: Every squat, smile, and stretch is a celebration of you. Let's age gracefully—one empowered movement at a time!

BEAUTY SLEEP: UNLOCKING THE SCIENCE OF SKIN-FRIENDLY SLEEP HABITS

Sleep is one of the most effective (and natural) anti-aging tools available. But did you know that how you sleep and what you sleep on can impact your skin just as much as the hours you spend resting? Let's dive into the science of sleep positioning, pillow fabrics, and how they influence skin health. By understanding these factors, you can make simple changes to keep your skin smoother, reduce wrinkles, and wake up looking refreshed.

The Side-Sleeping Dilemma: How Pressure Leads to Wrinkles

Sleeping on your side may feel cozy, but it can actually contribute to facial wrinkles over time. Here's why: when you lie on your side, your face presses against the pillow, creating friction and pressure. This pressure compresses the skin, particularly around delicate areas like the eyes, cheeks, and forehead. Over time, repetitive compression causes "sleep lines" to form —fine lines and wrinkles that deepen with age.

The Science Behind It:

- **Collagen Breakdown**: Side-sleeping compresses the skin, weakening collagen fibers over time. Collagen is essential for skin's elasticity, and when it breaks down, the skin loses its ability to "bounce back," resulting in visible lines.
- **Circulation Impact**: Prolonged pressure disrupts blood flow to the skin in that area, which can reduce oxygen and nutrient delivery, slowing down cell repair and renewal processes.
- **Skin Folds**: Side-sleeping positions the face against the pillow, causing folds in the skin. These repetitive folds can lead to permanent wrinkles, especially as collagen production slows with age.

Solution:

- **Switch to Back Sleeping**: This position distributes weight evenly across the face, reducing pressure points and helping to prevent compression lines. For added comfort, try a pillow designed to support back sleeping.

Silk vs. Cotton Pillowcases: Understanding the Difference

The material of your pillowcase plays a surprisingly significant role in skin aging. While cotton is a popular and breathable fabric, it can be abrasive against the skin, causing friction. On the other hand, silk offers a smoother surface with less drag on the skin and hair.

Why Cotton May Not Be Ideal:

- **Friction and Tugging**: Cotton fibers, though soft, can cause micro-friction as you move during sleep. This friction gently tugs at the skin, which may contribute to stretching and pulling, especially on delicate facial skin.
- **Absorption of Moisture**: Cotton tends to absorb moisture from the skin and hair, drawing away your natural oils and potentially the skincare products applied before bed. This can leave the skin feeling dry and less hydrated by morning.

The Benefits of Silk:

- **Reduced Friction**: Silk's ultra-smooth surface glides over the skin, significantly reducing friction. This minimizes the risk of skin pulling, helping the skin retain its elasticity and reducing the likelihood of wrinkle formation.
- **Preservation of Skin Hydration**: Unlike cotton, silk doesn't absorb as much moisture, which means it won't pull your nighttime skincare products away from your face. This helps keep your skin hydrated throughout the night, allowing products like moisturizers and serums to work effectively.
- **Gentle on Hair**: Silk is also gentler on hair, reducing tangles, breakage, and frizz. So, if you're looking for a

way to maintain smoother skin and healthier hair, a silk pillowcase could be the answer.

Actionable Tips:

1. **Invest in a Silk Pillowcase**: Start with one or two silk pillowcases and alternate them with your cotton pillowcases. Silk is a long-lasting material, making it a worthy investment in your skincare routine.
2. **Combine with Moisturizing Night Care**: Since silk helps retain moisture, apply a hydrating moisturizer or serum before bed to maximize your skin's overnight hydration and repair.
3. **Try Back Sleeping with Silk**: To get the best results, combine back sleeping with a silk pillowcase. It may take a little time to adjust, but the benefits are worth it—your skin and hair will thank you!

Why Beauty Sleep Matters for Aging Gracefully

Think of sleep as your skin's overnight repair team. While you rest, your body works hard to replenish collagen, repair cell damage, and restore hydration levels. By optimizing your sleep habits and environment, you're giving your skin the best possible conditions to thrive.

So, embrace the power of beauty sleep—not just as an anti-aging strategy, but as a form of self-care. With these simple adjustments, you'll wake up each day looking refreshed, radiant, and ready to take on the world. After all, nothing beats the glow of well-rested skin!

EMBRACING NEW AGING INNOVATIONS

Aging gracefully isn't about fighting against time—it's about working with it and, sometimes, embracing the incredible possibilities that science offers. From breakthroughs in cellular health to wearable technologies that help us live smarter, these innovations are redefining what it means to age. Imagine being able to track your health with a smartwatch or using therapies that rejuvenate your body from within—sounds like science fiction, right? But it's happening, and these advancements are closer than you think.

Let's explore how these tools and therapies can empower us to not just age gracefully but thrive while doing so.

Telomere Therapy: A New Frontier in Longevity

Imagine your DNA as a shoelace, with telomeres acting as the protective caps at the ends, much like the plastic tips that keep shoelaces from fraying. Telomeres play a critical role in maintaining cellular health by protecting your chromosomes. But as we age, telomeres naturally shorten with each cell division, and when they become too short, cells stop functioning efficiently or die. This is one of the key processes behind aging.

What Is Telomere Therapy?

Telomere therapy is a revolutionary concept aimed at slowing, stopping, or even reversing telomere shortening. This therapy focuses on extending cellular vitality by either activating an enzyme called telomerase (which rebuilds telomeres) or using advanced genetic tools to maintain telomere length.

Why Telomeres Matter:

- **Aging and Cellular Health:** Shortened telomeres are linked to cellular aging, tissue deterioration, and age-related diseases.
- **Disease Prevention:** Telomere therapy could reduce the risk of chronic conditions like heart disease, diabetes, and certain cancers by improving cellular repair and resilience.

- **Longevity and Vitality:** Supporting telomere health preserves physical and cognitive functions, keeping us energized and thriving as we age.

The Science and Future Potential:

Telomere therapy may soon include methods like telomerase activation (stimulating the natural enzyme to rebuild telomeres) or gene editing tools like CRISPR to repair telomeres directly. Nutritional supplements, such as TA-65 derived from the herb Astragalus, also show promise in supporting telomere health, though more research is needed.

What You Can Do Now to Protect Telomeres:

While telomere therapy continues to develop, you can take practical steps today to slow telomere shortening:

- Embrace an anti-inflammatory diet rich in antioxidants (think berries, greens, and nuts).
- Incorporate regular exercise to preserve cellular health.
- Manage stress levels with mindfulness, yoga, or meditation.
- Prioritize quality sleep, as it supports cellular repair.

Telomere therapy may sound like science fiction, but the research is advancing rapidly, bringing us closer to a future where we can prolong vitality and slow the visible signs of aging.

Genetic and Cellular Therapies: Rewriting the Aging Blueprint

Imagine if your body could repair itself, restoring vitality and health at the cellular level. Genetic and cellular therapies are making that dream a reality. These cutting-edge advancements focus on repairing damaged cells and targeting the genes responsible for aging, aiming to slow down the process from the inside out.

- **Why It's Exciting**: These therapies aren't just about looking younger—they could potentially enhance immunity, energy levels, and even mental clarity. For example, genetic therapies might one day repair age-related damage to our DNA, giving us a second chance to feel vibrant and strong.
- **A Real-Life Connection**: I often think about how these advancements might change life for my children. Imagine a world where they don't just live longer but live better—spending more active years with their families and pursuing their dreams with full energy.

Stem Cell and Telomere Therapy: Protecting Your Cellular Clock

Stem cells and telomeres play a crucial role in how our bodies age. Telomeres, the protective "caps" at the ends of our DNA, shorten as we age, reducing our cells' ability to repair themselves. Stem cells, on the other hand, have the potential to regenerate damaged tissues. New therapies aim to lengthen telomeres and harness the power of stem cells to extend cellular vitality.

- **What This Means for You**: Think of telomeres like the tips of your shoelaces—when they fray, the laces (your DNA) don't function as well. Therapies targeting telomere health could help keep your "laces" intact, protecting your cells and tissues from premature aging.
- **What You Can Do Now**: While these therapies are still developing, you can support your telomeres today with simple lifestyle changes. Exercise, stress management, and a diet rich in antioxidants can slow telomere shortening, helping you feel stronger and more resilient.

Wearable Health Technology: Your Personal Health Coach

Gone are the days of waiting for your next doctor's appointment to know how you're doing. Wearable health technology is bringing personalized wellness right to your wrist, helping you track everything from sleep patterns to hormonal fluctuations.

- **Why It Matters**: These devices aren't just gadgets—they're tools that empower you to take charge of your health. Imagine being able to monitor your stress levels during a busy workday or track your sleep quality after trying a new bedtime routine. By giving you real-time data, wearable tech makes it easier to spot patterns and make adjustments that improve your well-being.
- **A Personal Story**: When I first got a fitness tracker, I was skeptical. But after seeing how my stress levels spiked during certain times of the day, I realized I needed to prioritize moments of calm. Whether it's a five-minute meditation or a quick walk outside, having that insight has helped me feel more balanced—and yes, my skin has thanked me for it!

THE BRIGHT FUTURE OF AGING GRACEFULLY

As I look at these advancements, I can't help but feel a mix of awe and hope. Imagine a future where my daughter, decades from now, could use therapies to maintain her health and energy—or where I could track my body's needs as easily as checking my phone. These innovations aren't just about defying aging; they're about giving us the tools to live fully and confidently.

But remember, these breakthroughs are just the icing on the cake. The foundation of graceful aging remains in our hands: nurturing our bodies, practicing mindfulness, and cherishing the connections that bring joy and meaning to our lives.

So, as we embrace these exciting possibilities, let's also hold on to the timeless truths. Aging isn't something to fear—it's a journey of growth, resilience, and endless discovery. With the right mix of science, self-care, and heart, we can step boldly into the future and make every year our best one yet.

CONCLUSION: AGING GRACEFULLY, LIVING VIBRANTLY

Aging gracefully is not simply about routines or rituals—it's about embracing life with vitality, resilience, and purpose. It's about choosing to celebrate the unique beauty that each season of life brings while nourishing your body, mind, and soul. Every wrinkle, every laugh line, and every strand of gray hair tells the story of a life lived fully—a tapestry woven with experiences, wisdom, and strength.

From staying hydrated and savoring nourishing foods to exploring the cutting edge of scientific innovations, every step you take supports a more vibrant, radiant life. These aren't just habits; they're acts of self-love that honor the incredible person you are and the powerful legacy you're creating.

As women, we often carry the weight of many roles—nurturers, leaders, dreamers. But aging gracefully reminds us that it's okay, even necessary, to nurture ourselves. It's an invitation to let go of perfection, embrace authenticity, and prioritize what truly matters: our health, our happiness, and our inner glow.

Aging isn't about losing; it's about gaining—wisdom that sharpens your perspective, experiences that enrich your soul, and confidence that radiates from within. It's about transforming the fear of "getting older" into the freedom to live boldly, laugh often, and grow beautifully.

So, let this be your call to action: approach each year with intention, grace, and a dash of courage. Celebrate yourself—not in spite of aging, but because of it. Let your journey of graceful aging be a source of inspiration to those around you, a reminder that beauty is not about resisting time but embracing it with open arms.

Here's to living vibrantly, thriving boldly, and aging gracefully —because every chapter of your life deserves to be extraordinary.

CHAPTER 17

WHAT'S REALLY IN YOUR MAKEUP? A GUIDE TO BEAUTY CHOICES FOR HEALTH-CONSCIOUS WOMEN

THE TRUTH ABOUT COSMETICS—ARE THEY HELPING OR HARMING YOUR SKIN?

MAKEUP MATTERS—MORE THAN SKIN DEEP

Makeup is a staple for many of us—it's that swipe of lipstick before heading out the door, a little blush to brighten our day, or the confidence boost from a bold eyeliner. Whether it's for a casual outing or a big event, makeup often feels like an extension of who we are. But let's be honest: how often do we stop to think about what's actually in the products we're putting on our skin?

I'll admit it—I used to pick makeup based on three things: how it looked, whether it was on sale, and if someone said it worked miracles. A foundation that promised a "radiant glow"? I was in. An irresistible lipstick in the perfect shade of red? Sold! But my excitement was often short-lived. I vividly remember one foundation that left me with breakouts after just a few uses, far from the glow I had envisioned. Then there was the eyeliner that a friend swore by—except it made my eyes water so much I couldn't keep it on for more than an hour. And don't get me started on the matte lipstick that left my lips looking and feeling like sandpaper.

It was frustrating—and eye-opening. These weren't isolated incidents; they were a wake-up call. I began to question why certain products caused such reactions. Was it just my skin being "sensitive," or was there more to the story? Spoiler alert: it was the ingredients.

The truth is, what we put on our skin matters. Our skin is not just a protective barrier; it's an active organ that absorbs much of what we apply to it. Harsh chemicals, synthetic fragrances, and questionable preservatives can do more harm than we realize over time, from irritation and dryness to potentially long-term health effects.

This chapter is about looking beyond the pretty packaging and marketing buzzwords. It's about becoming a more informed consumer, empowering yourself with knowledge to make better beauty choices. Together, we'll explore why ingredients matter, how to identify harmful chemicals, and what to look for in products that truly prioritize your health. Because real beauty isn't just about how makeup makes you look—it's about how it makes you feel, inside and out.

So, let's dive in, redefine what "beautiful" means in your makeup bag, and create a routine that loves your skin as much as you do.

SECTION 1: WHY MAKEUP INGREDIENTS MATTER

Makeup is more than just a way to enhance your features; it's a product you apply directly to your skin—and sometimes ingest unintentionally. Let's dive into the science of why being mindful of makeup ingredients is essential for your health, beauty, and confidence.

1. Lips: More Than Just a Pretty Pout

Lipstick might be your go-to for that pop of color, but did you know that whatever you swipe on your lips could end up inside your body? Studies have revealed that many lipsticks contain

heavy metals like lead and cadmium, which may accumulate over time. According to the Campaign for Safe Cosmetics, lead in lipstick doesn't just dry out your lips—it's also a neurotoxin that has no safe level of exposure.

What to Watch For:

- **Parabens and Petrochemicals**: These preservatives and synthetic ingredients can dry out your lips or irritate sensitive skin. Long-term exposure to parabens has been linked to hormone disruption.
- **Artificial Dyes**: Often derived from petroleum, these dyes may cause allergies or sensitivity in some people.

Safer Alternatives: Look for lipsticks with **natural oils** like coconut or castor oil, **beeswax**, or **vitamin E**, which can nourish and hydrate your lips. Brands offering **organic** or **plant-based pigments** are great options for safer, healthier lips.

Pro Tip: If your lipstick is making your lips feel dry or uncomfortable, it might be time to swap it out for a product with **clean ingredients**. Think of your lipstick not just as makeup but as skincare for your lips!

2. Foundation vs. Cushion Compact: The SPF Dilemma

Foundations and cushion compacts are the backbone of many beauty routines, but the added SPF in some products can be a double-edged sword. While these products provide lightweight coverage and sun protection, most don't deliver enough SPF for all-day coverage. Studies show that makeup with SPF often requires reapplication to maintain efficacy—and let's be honest, who reapplies foundation midday?

The Breakdown:

- **Foundation**: Provides fuller coverage but may clog pores if it contains talc or synthetic fillers.

- **Cushion Compact**: Perfect for a natural, dewy finish but often has SPF levels that need reinforcement.

Best Practice: Use a dedicated **broad-spectrum sunscreen** (SPF 30 or higher) under your foundation or cushion compact. SPF in makeup should be seen as a bonus, not as your main source of sun protection.

3. False Lashes and Glue: The Good, the Bad, and the Lashes

False lashes can transform your look in seconds, but their glue can often contain **formaldehyde**—a chemical known to irritate the skin and eyes, and even weaken your natural lashes over time. Frequent use of these glues can lead to redness, lash fallout, or even allergic reactions.

What to Avoid:

- **Formaldehyde and Latex**: These are common irritants that can cause sensitivities.
- **Fragrances**: Artificial scents in lash adhesives can irritate the delicate eye area.

Safer Options: Choose **formaldehyde-free** and **latex-free glues** or switch to **magnetic lashes**. Magnetic lashes use tiny magnets to stay in place, avoiding the need for adhesive altogether. If you prefer using glue, give your natural lashes a break between applications to keep them healthy.

4. Eyeliner: A Close-Up Look at Ingredients Near the Eyes

Eyeliner can define your eyes beautifully, but it's applied close to one of the most sensitive parts of your body. Some liners contain **parabens**, **synthetic dyes**, and **preservatives** that may irritate your eyes.

What to Look For:

- **Hypoallergenic Liners**: Especially important if you have sensitive skin or wear contact lenses.
- **Natural Pigments**: Opt for liners that use mineral pigments or plant-based ingredients for color.

SECTION 2: MAKING SAFER, SMARTER MAKEUP CHOICES

1. Concealer, Bronzer, Highlighter, and Contour Products

These products often sit on your skin all day, so choosing options with skin-loving ingredients is essential. Many powders and creams contain **talc**, which can clog pores or cause dryness.

Tips for Smarter Choices:

- **Mineral-Based Products**: Look for mica, zinc oxide, and titanium dioxide, which provide lightweight coverage while being gentle on the skin.
- **Nourishing Ingredients**: Products with **shea butter**, **aloe vera**, or **jojoba oil** can hydrate and soothe your skin during wear.

2. Ingredients to Avoid and Ingredients to Embrace

Avoid:

- **Parabens**: Preservatives that mimic estrogen and may disrupt hormones.
- **Phthalates**: Often found in fragrances and linked to hormonal imbalances.
- **Artificial Fragrances**: These can cause irritation, especially for sensitive skin.
- **Talc**: Can clog pores and has raised concerns about contamination with asbestos.

Embrace:

- **Vitamin E**: An antioxidant that soothes and protects the skin.
- **Jojoba Oil**: Mimics the skin's natural oils and provides hydration without clogging pores.
- **Green Tea Extract**: Fights inflammation and offers antioxidant protection.
- **Hyaluronic Acid**: Hydrates and plumps the skin, making it a great addition to makeup.

FINAL THOUGHTS

Understanding what's in your makeup is more than just a trend—it's a form of self-care. By choosing products with safe, nourishing ingredients, you're not only enhancing your beauty but also protecting your health. Remember, beauty is skin deep, but health is deeper. Let your makeup be a reflection of the care and respect you have for your body.

NATURAL MAKEUP REMOVERS: GENTLE AND NOURISHING OPTIONS

We all know the feeling—coming home after a long day, ready to unwind, only to face the tedious task of taking off your makeup. But what if this nightly ritual could double as a pampering skincare moment? With natural makeup removers, you can clean your skin while nourishing it, leaving your face refreshed, hydrated, and glowing. Here are some tried-and-true natural methods to remove makeup that are gentle on your skin and effective for even waterproof products.

Coconut Oil

Coconut oil is a multitasking powerhouse. Rich in fatty acids, it moisturizes and protects your skin, while its antibacterial properties help heal and prevent infections. As a makeup remover, coconut oil effectively dissolves all types of makeup, including waterproof mascara.

To use:

- Warm up solid coconut oil until it becomes liquid.
- Apply it to your face with a cotton ball or your fingertips, and gently massage in circular motions.
- Rinse thoroughly with warm water, then follow up with your regular cleanser to avoid clogged pores.

Pro tip: Opt for organic, cold-pressed coconut oil to ensure you're getting all its nutrients intact. However, if you have sensitive skin prone to allergic reactions, perform a patch test first to avoid irritation.

Olive Oil

Another kitchen favorite, olive oil, is a fantastic natural option for breaking down even the most stubborn makeup. Its oil-attracts-oil properties make it especially effective for waterproof mascara. Additionally, olive oil contains vitamin E and antioxidants that nourish and protect your skin, leaving it soft and hydrated.

To use:

- Pour a small amount onto a cotton pad.
- Gently rub it over your face and eyelashes in circular motions.
- Wash your face afterward with your usual cleanser to remove any oily residue.

Bonus: Olive oil's antioxidants combat free radicals, while its oleic acid hydrates and smooths fine lines, making it a skincare ally.

Jojoba Oil

Jojoba oil is often hailed as one of the best natural makeup removers—and for good reason! Its chemical structure closely mimics your skin's natural sebum, making it an excellent option for all skin types, including oily or acne-prone skin. Jojoba oil effectively dissolves makeup without clogging pores and offers added hydration and protection with its rich content of vitamin E and antioxidants.

To use:

- Apply a few drops of jojoba oil to a cotton pad or your fingertips.
- Massage gently over your face and eyes to loosen makeup.
- Rinse with warm water or use a damp cloth to wipe away residue, then follow up with your favorite cleanser for a fresh finish.

Why it's a winner: Jojoba oil is non-comedogenic, hypoaller-genic, and packed with anti-inflammatory properties, making it gentle and safe for daily use. It leaves your skin soft, balanced, and nourished without feeling greasy.

By incorporating natural oils like coconut, olive, or jojoba into your makeup removal routine, you're not only cleansing your skin but also infusing it with nutrients that enhance its health and glow. Whether you're winding down after a long day or indulging in a little self-care, these gentle yet effective options make makeup removal a ritual to look forward to!

Milk

Yes, milk! This humble fridge staple is a surprising yet effective natural makeup remover. The lactic acid in milk gently exfoli-ates while breaking down makeup and dirt. It also hydrates and soothes the skin, making it perfect for those with dry or sensi-tive skin.

To use:

- Soak a cotton pad in milk (preferably whole milk for its fat content).
- Swipe it across your face and let the residue sit for a few minutes before rinsing it off.

Pro tip: For extra hydration, leave the milk on overnight (if you're comfortable) and wake up to supple, glowing skin.

Sugar Scrub

For those looking to combine makeup removal with exfoliation, a sugar scrub is the perfect solution. Sugar gently buffs away dead skin cells and removes impurities lodged deep in your pores while promoting blood circulation for that radiant glow.

To use:

- Mix equal parts sugar with olive oil, honey, or another carrier oil to create a paste.
- Massage the scrub into your skin in gentle circular motions.
- Rinse thoroughly with warm water to reveal baby-soft skin.

This DIY scrub is not just a remover—it's a rejuvenating treat for your face, leaving it cleansed and radiant.

Choosing the Right Makeup Remover

If you prefer store-bought makeup removers, look for products that are alcohol-free and formulated with nourishing ingredients like aloe vera, chamomile, or vitamin E. These are gentle on the delicate eye area and help prevent eyelash breakage. Avoid harsh removers with strong fragrances or astringents, as they can dry out your skin and irritate your eyes.

A NOURISHING FINAL NOTE

Your makeup removal routine doesn't have to feel like a chore. By choosing natural, nourishing options, you're not just cleansing your skin—you're pampering it. Whether you opt for coconut oil, olive oil, milk, or a DIY sugar scrub, these methods are gentle, effective, and kind to your skin.

So, the next time you're ready to wind down, let your makeup removal routine become a moment of self-care. Your skin—and lashes—will thank you!

SECTION 3: MAKEUP FOR THE HEALTH-CONSCIOUS: WHAT TO LOOK FOR AND WHERE TO START

Makeup is more than just a way to enhance your beauty—it's also a part of your self-care routine. For health-conscious women, selecting the right products means balancing beauty and wellness. Here's how to make mindful, skin-friendly choices without sacrificing style or performance.

1. Choosing "Clean" Brands

The beauty industry is brimming with options, but not all products are created equal. Clean beauty brands are a fantastic place to start for anyone looking to avoid harmful ingredients and embrace a more holistic approach.

What to Look For:

- **Paraben-Free**: Parabens are preservatives that may disrupt hormones. Opt for products that explicitly state they are paraben-free.
- **Sulfate-Free**: Sulfates can strip your skin of natural oils and cause irritation.
- **Cruelty-Free**: Support brands that don't test on animals.
- **Vegan**: Vegan products exclude any animal-derived

ingredients, which can be a great choice for ethical beauty lovers.

Tip: Researching brands ahead of time and reading ingredient lists can save you from buying products that don't align with your health priorities. Clean beauty stores or sections in major retailers make it easier to find curated options.

2. SPF and Sun Safety in Makeup

We've all seen makeup products that boast SPF benefits, but is it enough? While it's great that foundations, BB creams, and even powders now offer sun protection, they shouldn't replace a dedicated sunscreen.

Why Dedicated Sunscreen Matters:

- The amount of SPF in makeup is often insufficient for all-day protection.
- You would need to apply several layers of SPF makeup to achieve the recommended level of coverage, which isn't practical.

Best Practice:

- Use a broad-spectrum sunscreen with at least SPF 30 as your first layer before applying makeup.
- Think of SPF-infused makeup as a bonus layer of protection, especially for touch-ups during the day.

3. Maintaining Natural Lashes with Mascara

Mascara is a staple for many women, but it's important to choose formulas that enhance your lashes without causing damage. Traditional mascaras can sometimes dry out your lashes or make them brittle, so opting for nourishing options is key.

What to Look For:

- **Castor Oil**: This ingredient is known for its lash-conditioning properties, helping lashes grow stronger and fuller over time.
- **Biotin**: A form of vitamin B, biotin supports keratin production, which can improve lash health.
- **Gentle, Hypoallergenic Formulas**: Especially important if you have sensitive eyes.

Pro Tip: Avoid waterproof mascaras for everyday use—they're harder to remove, which can lead to lash breakage. Instead, save them for special occasions and opt for nourishing formulas for daily wear.

By being intentional about the makeup you choose, you're not only enhancing your beauty but also protecting and nourishing your skin and lashes. Start small by incorporating one or two clean beauty swaps into your routine, and over time, you'll build a collection of products that align with your values and keep your skin looking its best.

As we've explored, makeup is more than just a tool for enhancing beauty—it's an extension of self-care and personal expression. But the beauty world is constantly evolving, with exciting trends and innovations reshaping how we approach our makeup routines. From eco-conscious choices to skin-friendly formulations, today's trends are all about aligning beauty with health, mindfulness, and sustainability. Let's dive into some of the most inspiring holistic makeup trends that are making waves—and how they can fit seamlessly into your routine.

1. Skinimalism: Enhancing Natural Beauty

- **What It Is**: Skinimalism is all about embracing your natural skin texture and using minimal makeup for a fresh, radiant look. It's less about covering up imperfections and more about enhancing what you already have.

- **Why It's Trending**: Women are moving toward lighter, breathable makeup that lets their skin shine through.
- **Holistic Tip**: Use multi-purpose products like tinted moisturizers with SPF, cream blushes that double as lip color, or hydrating highlighters for a dewy finish.

2. Ayurvedic Makeup

- **What It Is**: Inspired by Ayurveda, this approach uses makeup infused with herbal and plant-based ingredients that are believed to balance your body's energy and improve overall health.
- **Examples**: Products infused with **turmeric** for its anti-inflammatory properties or **sandalwood** for its cooling effects on the skin.
- **Why It's Trending**: Ayurvedic beauty blends ancient wisdom with modern convenience, offering health-conscious women makeup that nourishes while it beautifies.

3. Refillable and Sustainable Packaging

- **What It Is**: Beauty brands are introducing refillable makeup products to reduce waste. Think lipstick cases or compact powders that you can replenish without throwing away the container.
- **Why It's Trending**: Environmental consciousness is growing, and women want beauty products that reflect their commitment to sustainability.
- **Holistic Tip**: Look for brands offering biodegradable, recyclable, or refillable packaging. Supporting these products is an act of self-care for both you and the planet.

4. Microbiome-Friendly Makeup

- **What It Is**: This trend focuses on makeup that supports your skin's microbiome—a collection of beneficial bacteria that keeps your skin healthy.
- **Why It's Trending**: With the growing awareness of gut health's connection to skin health, products are now designed to maintain a balanced microbiome, reducing breakouts and irritation.
- **Key Ingredients**: **Probiotics, prebiotics, and postbiotics**.
- **Holistic Tip**: Pair these makeup products with a balanced skincare routine to maximize benefits.

6. DIY or Customizable Makeup

- **What It Is**: Some brands offer DIY kits or customizable formulas so women can create their own makeup shades and textures using natural ingredients.
- **Why It's Trending**: It empowers women to control what goes into their makeup while allowing for personal creativity.
- **Holistic Tip**: Explore kits with organic pigments and natural bases to create a truly tailored beauty routine.

7. Blue Light Protection in Makeup

- **What It Is**: With increased screen time, makeup with blue-light-blocking ingredients is becoming more popular. These products claim to protect your skin from the effects of prolonged exposure to digital devices.
- **Key Ingredients**: Zinc oxide, niacinamide, and antioxidants like vitamin C.
- **Why It's Trending**: As remote work and online activity grow, this innovation is becoming essential for modern lifestyles.

- **Holistic Tip**: Combine these products with screen time management and nighttime skin detox routines for added protection.

8. Vegan Makeup Brushes

- **What It Is**: Makeup brushes made with synthetic bristles rather than animal-derived ones, offering an ethical and cruelty-free alternative.
- **Why It's Trending**: Vegan brushes are more affordable, hypoallergenic, and aligned with the values of ethical beauty.
- **Holistic Tip**: Clean your brushes regularly to maintain skin health and extend their lifespan.

CONCLUSION: BEAUTY CHOICES THAT EMPOWER AND UPLIFT

Choosing makeup thoughtfully isn't just about what we put on our faces—it's about embracing our worth, prioritizing our well-being, and redefining beauty as a reflection of self-care and authenticity. Makeup has the power to enhance, but the real glow comes from the confidence and care we pour into ourselves.

By taking a few moments to research ingredients, support brands that align with our values, and choose products that nurture our skin, we're not just investing in beauty; we're investing in health and empowerment. Think of it as an act of self-love—one that extends beyond appearances and into the way we value and treat ourselves every day.

Just as we've learned to read the labels on our food and embrace nourishing choices for our bodies, we can apply the same care to our makeup routines. After all, beauty is not just about how we look; it's about how we feel. It's about being informed, intentional, and inspired to make choices that align with the radiant, vibrant women we are.

So, the next time you reach for that lipstick or foundation, let it be a reminder: you deserve products that uplift you, inside and out. Let your makeup be a celebration of your unique beauty, a tool to express your individuality, and a means to empower yourself with every swipe and shade.

Because when we approach beauty mindfully and holistically, we're not just painting faces; we're honoring the incredible women we are—and that's the kind of glow that lasts a lifetime.

CHAPTER 18

AROMATHERAPY

A NATURAL BOOST FOR YOUR MIND, BODY, AND SPIRIT

MORE THAN JUST A PRETTY SCENT

Aromatherapy isn't just about creating a luxurious ambiance or indulging in a fancy spa treatment—it's a holistic practice rooted in centuries of tradition. Using natural plant extracts, known as essential oils, aromatherapy offers powerful benefits for your mind, body, and spirit. It's a gentle yet transformative way to improve your well-being, reduce stress, and even enhance your beauty routine—all without requiring hours of your time.

You've probably experienced it before: walking into a spa and being instantly enveloped in the calming scent of lavender or the invigorating aroma of eucalyptus. That moment of peace isn't just in your head—it's the science of aromatherapy at work. Now imagine bringing that same calm or energy boost into your daily life, no spa appointment required. Whether you're facing sleepless nights, an overwhelming to-do list, or simply seeking a small moment of self-care, aromatherapy can become your go-to solution.

A PERSONAL JOURNEY INTO AROMATHERAPY

As a working mother balancing a career, family, and personal well-being, I found myself searching for ways to bring calm into my chaotic life. That's when I stumbled upon aromatherapy—not as a luxury, but as a lifeline.

It all started with a small bottle of lavender essential oil. I diffused it one evening when my kids were restless from colds, and within minutes, the atmosphere shifted. Lavender didn't just help them sleep better; it calmed my frazzled nerves, too. Soon, eucalyptus became a household staple for clearing up sinuses, and peppermint gave me an energizing lift during those mid-afternoon slumps (when even coffee wasn't cutting it).

But aromatherapy's magic isn't just about nice smells. It's about how those scents interact with our bodies and minds. Lavender, for example, became my multitasking hero—soothing burns, helping with insect bites, calming eczema, and even reducing stress. Diffusing it at night turned our home into a sanctuary of relaxation, where everyone—including the kids—could sleep more peacefully. It was more than a routine; it became a ritual of care and connection.

Through my journey, I learned that aromatherapy is a beautiful blend of science and soul. Each essential oil offers unique benefits, and discovering how they fit into my life felt empowering. From creating a calming bedtime ritual to enhancing family wellness, aromatherapy became my secret weapon for finding balance amidst life's chaos.

HOW AROMATHERAPY WORKS: THE SCIENCE BEHIND THE SCENTS

Aromatherapy harnesses the power of essential oils extracted from plants to enhance physical, emotional, and mental well-being. These potent oils work by interacting with your body in remarkable ways, and understanding how they function can help you use them more effectively.

When you inhale an essential oil, its aromatic molecules travel through your nose and stimulate your olfactory system, which is directly linked to the brain's limbic system. This part of the brain governs emotions, memories, and even vital functions like heart rate and stress responses. Think of it as a direct line between what you smell and how you feel.

For example, breathing in lavender oil is more than just enjoying a pleasant fragrance—it engages the limbic system to promote relaxation and reduce stress. I like to call it my "chill in a bottle." Feeling overwhelmed or restless? A whiff of lavender can signal your brain to release serotonin, helping to calm the chaos and bring you back to balance.

Aromatherapy isn't just about relaxation, though. If you're struggling to focus or need an energy lift, invigorating scents like citrus oils (orange or lemon) can do the trick. These bright aromas stimulate your nervous system, enhancing concentration and boosting your mood—no triple espresso required. On days when your immune system needs extra support, oils like eucalyptus or peppermint come to the rescue. Not only do they clear your sinuses, but they also create a refreshing sensation that instantly makes you feel more awake and alive.

When applied topically, essential oils can also benefit the body through absorption. Mixed with carrier oils, they penetrate the skin and work their magic on a deeper level. For instance, tea tree oil is known for its antimicrobial properties, making it great for acne or minor cuts, while rosemary oil can help ease muscle tension after a long day.

Incorporating aromatherapy into your life is like having a personalized wellness toolkit. Whether you need calm, focus, or a breath of fresh air—literally—there's an essential oil for that. It's a natural, accessible way to nurture your mind, body, and spirit.

CHOOSING THE RIGHT ESSENTIAL OILS: A GUIDE TO YOUR AROMATHERAPY TOOLKIT

With countless essential oils out there, picking the right one can feel a bit overwhelming. But don't worry—it's simpler than it seems. Choosing essential oils comes down to your personal needs, preferences, and how your body and mind respond to different scents. Let's explore some popular essential oils and their incredible benefits, with a dash of personality to make your selection process fun and engaging!

Lavender: The Jack-of-All-Trades

Lavender is the go-to essential oil for a reason—it does it all. Feeling stressed? Lavender has your back. Struggling to sleep? A few drops of lavender will lull you into dreamland. Got a burn or a bug bite? Yep, lavender to the rescue! It's basically the Swiss Army knife of essential oils, perfect for relaxation, skin healing, and even soothing eczema. If you're new to aromatherapy, lavender is a must-have in your starter kit.

Peppermint: Your Energizing BFF

Need an energy boost but don't want another cup of coffee? Peppermint is here to save the day. Known for its cooling, refreshing scent, peppermint improves focus, relieves headaches, and can even soothe sore muscles. Just one sniff, and you'll feel like you can tackle anything—whether it's a pile of paperwork or a mountain of laundry. Bonus: It's a lifesaver during hot flashes, offering instant relief when you need it most.

Eucalyptus: The Breath of Fresh Air

If your sinuses are screaming for help, eucalyptus is the essential oil equivalent of a deep, cleansing breath. It's amazing for respiratory health, clearing congestion, and even boosting your immune system. A few drops in a diffuser can transform your room into a personal spa, complete with that "just breathe" vibe. Trust me, your lungs will thank you.

Tea Tree: Nature's Tiny Warrior

Tea tree oil is a powerhouse for skin health. Whether you're battling acne, a fungal infection, or a minor cut, this antibacterial, antifungal, and antiviral oil is like having a little warrior on your bathroom shelf. Dab it on pesky breakouts, or mix it with a carrier oil to soothe itchy skin—it's a multitasker you'll want in your arsenal.

Rose: A Romantic Elixir

Rose oil isn't just about smelling like a bouquet—it's an emotional well-being booster. Known for reducing anxiety and promoting skin elasticity, rose oil helps you feel grounded and luxurious all at once. Whether you're pampering yourself with a facial or just need a moment of calm, this floral favorite is pure indulgence.

Ylang Ylang: The Mood Balancer

If life feels a bit chaotic (and let's be honest, when doesn't it?), ylang ylang can help you find your emotional balance. Its rich, floral scent is perfect for calming anger, easing anxiety, and lifting your spirits. Think of it as your emotional support oil for those moments when the Wi-Fi crashes or the kids suddenly remember a forgotten school project at bedtime.

How to Choose the Right Oil for You

Let your intuition (and your nose) guide you. Essential oils can evoke unique emotional responses, so if a particular scent makes you feel good, it's the right one for you. But fair warning: don't try to sniff every oil at once, or you might end up feeling like you walked into an overzealous perfume shop.

If you're still unsure, start with a basic toolkit:

- **Lavender** for relaxation and sleep.
- **Peppermint** for focus and energy.
- **Eucalyptus** for respiratory health.
- **Tea Tree** for skin care.
- **Rose** for emotional balance.
- **Ylang Ylang** for mood regulation.

And remember, this isn't a one-size-fits-all journey. Play around with combinations to find your personal favorites. You might just discover a signature blend that lifts your spirits, clears your mind, and nurtures your body. Aromatherapy is all about tuning into what you need, so have fun experimenting!

THE POWER OF AROMATHERAPY IN EVERYDAY LIFE

Picture this: It's the end of a long day. Deadlines were relentless, your kids are locked in a passionate debate over homework logistics, and tomorrow's to-do list already feels like a mountain. You could collapse onto the couch and scroll mindlessly through your phone, sure. Or—stay with me here—you could reach for a bottle of lavender essential oil, close your eyes, and take a few deep, soul-soothing breaths.

Feel the difference?

Aromatherapy isn't reserved for luxurious spa days or the rare moments when you "feel fancy." It's a simple, accessible way to reset, manage stress, and invite a little calm into the chaos of daily life. It's like a quiet superpower you can wield anytime, anywhere.

Imagine diffusing eucalyptus in the kitchen while whipping up dinner or adding a few drops of lavender to your bath to melt away the day's tension. Better yet, keep a rollerball of energizing peppermint oil in your bag for those mid-afternoon slumps. It's as easy as reaching for dry shampoo on a hectic morning—but for your mind, body, and spirit.

Aromatherapy isn't just about scents; it's about reclaiming moments of peace and balance in the middle of life's busyness. Think of it as your personal self-care toolkit—ready to help you reset, breathe, and face whatever comes your way.

AROMATHERAPY IN CLINICAL SETTINGS

Did you know essential oils are making their way into hospitals and clinical settings? That's right—it's not just for yoga studios and day spas anymore. Lavender, for example, is often used to help pre-surgery patients reduce stress and promote relaxation. Similarly, peppermint oil is gaining attention for managing nausea and mild pain, offering a natural alternative in certain medical treatments. Tea tree oil, renowned for its antibacterial properties, has even been utilized in some cases to combat infections like MRSA.

This isn't just anecdotal evidence—research backs the calming, therapeutic effects of essential oils when used appropriately. It's like a hospital-approved dose of serenity, proving that even in clinical environments, nature has a role to play in healing and wellness.

The Benefits of Sauna and Essential Oils

Now, let's take the relaxation factor up a notch by pairing aromatherapy with another time-tested wellness ritual: the sauna. If you haven't experienced the magic of a sauna session with essential oils, you're in for a treat.

Here's the science: the heat from a sauna opens your pores, allowing essential oils to deeply penetrate the skin. Simultaneously, the steam carries the aroma into your respiratory system, helping you breathe more freely and amplifying the calming or energizing effects of the oils. It's like a workout for your skin while your mind takes a peaceful retreat.

According to Dr. Berg, a respected voice in holistic wellness, the benefits of saunas extend beyond relaxation. They help detoxify the skin, boost circulation, alleviate stress, and even support weight loss. When combined with essential oils like eucalyptus for respiratory support or lavender for relaxation, the experience transforms into a full-body rejuvenation session.

Imagine stepping out of the sauna feeling refreshed, lighter, and more centered—like your skin just did yoga while your brain meditated. Whether you're a sauna enthusiast or a curious newbie, adding essential oils elevates this timeless practice into a luxurious, healing ritual that leaves you glowing inside and out.

Incorporating Aromatherapy into Your Routine

Aromatherapy is a simple yet powerful tool to enhance your daily life. Its versatility means there's something for everyone and every moment. Here are a few ways to weave the magic of essential oils into your routine:

- **Morning Boost**: Start your day with a burst of energy by diffusing peppermint or citrus oils like orange or lemon. These uplifting scents wake up your senses and improve focus—like sunshine in a bottle without the caffeine crash.
- **Midday Stress Relief**: Keep a small roller of lavender or bergamot oil in your bag. Apply it to your wrists, temples, or the back of your neck during stressful moments. It's like carrying a pocket-sized escape from the chaos of a grocery store meltdown or a never-ending to-do list.
- **Bedtime Relaxation**: Unwind after a long day by adding a few drops of lavender or chamomile oil to your pillow, diffuser, or a warm bath. These calming scents help ease you into a restful sleep. Warning: You might wake up feeling so refreshed that "snooze" becomes optional.

- **Post-Workout Revival**: After a workout or a long day on your feet, massage diluted peppermint or eucalyptus oil onto sore muscles. The cooling, invigorating sensation is like a reward for your body—and it pairs beautifully with a yoga mat and a deep stretch.
- **Family Time**: Make aromatherapy a household affair! Let your kids pick the scent of the day for the diffuser—it's a fun way to get them involved and introduce some calm into your home (even if it's just for a few minutes). Plus, a home that smells of lavender is a home that feels like a hug.

CONCLUSION: A BREATH OF BALANCE AND BEAUTY

Aromatherapy isn't just a fleeting wellness trend; it's a time-honored practice that invites balance, healing, and joy into your everyday life. Whether it's a burst of peppermint to jumpstart your morning, lavender to ease you into sweet dreams, or eucalyptus to energize your post-workout recovery, essential oils have a way of transforming ordinary moments into extraordinary ones.

The beauty of aromatherapy is its accessibility—it doesn't require expensive equipment or hours of effort, just a few drops of nature's magic. So, why not take a moment today to breathe deeply, embrace the scents that soothe your soul, and let aromatherapy remind you that self-care is never selfish?

Your mind, body, and spirit deserve this gift. Because when you feel good, you radiate that goodness to everyone around you. So go ahead, take that first breath—your journey to a more balanced and beautiful life begins here.

CHAPTER 19

AI (ARTIFICIAL INTELLIGENCE) IN BEAUTY AND WELLNESS

YOUR SMARTEST (AND MOST HELPFUL) COMPANION FOR HEALTH & RADIANCE

THE NEW BEST FRIEND YOU DIDN'T KNOW YOU NEEDED

Let's face it—life is busy. Whether you're juggling a career, raising kids, or simply trying to carve out a sliver of "me time" (what even is that?), the to-do list never seems to end. But what if you didn't have to do it all alone? Enter Artificial Intelligence (AI)—your tech-savvy companion in beauty, wellness, and everyday life.

Imagine this: a virtual assistant that reminds you to reapply sunscreen, plans family trips, curates your skincare routine, and even suggests activities to keep your kids entertained. Sounds futuristic? The future is here, and AI is changing the game.

WHY AI IS EVERY BUSY WOMAN'S SECRET WEAPON

We're already using AI in ways we may not even realize—from asking Alexa to play music to letting Google Maps guide us. But AI is now stepping into the beauty and wellness world, offering tailored solutions to make our lives easier, more efficient, and a little more fabulous.

For busy women, AI acts like the friend who always knows what to do, whether it's recommending a foundation that matches your skin tone perfectly or finding kid-friendly activities for the weekend. It's not just technology—it's a lifeline for managing the chaos of modern life.

AI IN BEAUTY: SKINCARE MEETS SCIENCE

Personalized Skincare: A Revolution in Beauty

Gone are the days of guessing which products work for your skin. AI-powered tools like L'Oréal Perso, OKU Personal Skin Coach, and YouCam Makeup analyze your skin and provide personalized recommendations.

- **How It Works:** Snap a selfie or use a scanning device to evaluate hydration levels, dark spots, fine lines, and redness. Based on the analysis, these apps suggest products or routines tailored to your unique needs.
- **Why It's a Game-Changer:** Instead of trial-and-error shopping, you'll get accurate, science-backed advice, saving time, money, and frustration.

Smart Sunscreen Reminders

Ever forget to reapply sunscreen during a busy day? Apps like QSun use UV exposure data to remind you when it's time to reapply SPF. It's like having a sun-care coach in your pocket, ensuring your skin stays protected.

AI-Driven Wearables: Beauty on the Go

Wearables like REDUIT are taking skincare to the next level. Using ultrasonic diffusion, they deliver active ingredients directly to your skin, maximizing absorption and minimizing waste. Imagine having a high-tech facial at home whenever you need it.

AI-Powered Hair Care: Tailored Solutions for Healthier Hair

Caring for your hair can feel like navigating a maze of products and promises—especially if you're dealing with dryness, breakage, or hair thinning. This is where AI-driven tools come to the rescue, offering personalized insights that take the guesswork out of hair care. By analyzing your scalp and hair using advanced imaging technology, these tools can pinpoint issues like hydration levels, scalp health, and even early signs of hair loss.

Here's how it works: some apps use AI-powered scalp imaging to assess the condition of your hair and provide tailored recommendations. Whether it's identifying the best treatments, suggesting products suited to your unique needs, or offering simple lifestyle tweaks, these tools make it easier to care for your hair. The real advantage? Many platforms track your progress over time, allowing you to see if your routine is working and adjust as needed.

There are apps, like **HairAI**, that focus on diagnostics rather than selling specific products, making them ideal for those who want unbiased insights. Meanwhile, brands like HairMax and Shiseido's AI Mirror are examples of tools that combine cutting-edge technology with personalized solutions. If you're exploring options, consider platforms that prioritize analysis and tracking over product sales, giving you greater control and flexibility in choosing the right approach for your hair.

For women managing hair thinning, these tools can be life-changing. They empower you to make data-driven decisions about your routine and provide reassurance that your efforts are making a difference. Whether you're optimizing your current care or addressing specific concerns, AI-driven hair care tools offer the support you need to nurture healthier, more vibrant hair.

AI IN WELLNESS: YOUR DIGITAL LIFE COACH

Fitness and Recovery Tailored to You

Wearables like Fitbit, WHOOP, and Apple Watch don't just count steps—they analyze sleep patterns, monitor stress levels, and even predict recovery times after workouts.

- **New Trends:** AI-powered fitness apps now recommend the best time to exercise based on your energy levels, helping you avoid burnout and stay consistent.

Mental Wellness at Your Fingertips

Feeling stressed? AI apps like Calm and Headspace offer guided meditations tailored to your mood. For more interactive support, platforms like Replika provide virtual life coaching to help you navigate emotions and build resilience.

AI FOR FAMILY LIFE: YOUR TIME-SAVING SUPERPOWER

Imagine skipping the endless scrolling and getting straight to what you need. Whether planning a family getaway, finding creative extracurricular activities for your kids, or exploring targeted workout plans, AI handles the research so you don't have to. It's like having a personal assistant who understands your unique needs and delivers results in minutes.

Need a workout plan that fits your schedule? AI can tailor exercises to your specific goals, like toning your core or slimming your waistline, while respecting your busy lifestyle. Want dinner ideas that match what's already in your fridge? Done. Planning a weekend trip? AI can generate an itinerary that balances fun for the kids and relaxation for you. It even helped me craft a detailed, step-by-step guide for my parents' citizenship application—a task that used to feel overwhelming but now feels manageable.

The best part? While AI does the legwork, you gain precious time to focus on what matters most—whether that's soaking in a well-deserved bath, diving into a good book, or simply savoring a moment of stillness. It's the ultimate game-changer for women balancing it all.

Planning Family Adventures Made Easy

Planning a family trip can feel overwhelming, but AI apps like Google Trips and PackPoint simplify the process:

- Itinerary Planning: These tools suggest kid-friendly activities, restaurants, and must-see attractions based on your destination.
- Packing Lists: Apps like PackPoint create customized packing lists, ensuring you don't forget sunscreen for the beach or jackets for a chilly mountain escape.

Educational Fun for Kids

AI platforms like Khan Academy Kids and Photomath make learning interactive and engaging. Whether it's helping with homework or finding educational videos, AI turns screen time into quality time.

Meal Planning for Picky Eaters

Apps like Yummly and Mealime create meal plans tailored to your family's preferences and dietary needs. AI even sneaks in recipes that make veggies palatable for your pickiest eaters.

EMBRACING THE FUTURE: AI TRENDS IN BEAUTY AND WELLNESS

AI is constantly evolving, offering exciting innovations that feel straight out of a sci-fi movie:

- **SkinVision:** This app analyzes moles and spots for early signs of skin concerns, providing peace of mind for health-conscious women.
- **AI-Powered Spas:** High-tech facials now use AI to scan your skin and tailor treatments in real time.
- **Virtual Dermatologists:** Apps like Curology connect you with skincare experts who create custom treatments based on your unique needs.

Tech Detox and Using AI Wisely as Part of Digital Wellness

While AI is a powerful tool, it's not a replacement for intuition or human connection. Think of AI as an assistant—not the boss. Use its insights to enhance your decisions, but remember to trust your instincts and listen to your body.

As much as AI simplifies life—organizing schedules, curating skincare routines, and even supporting mental health—it's essential to recognize when technology crosses the line from helpful to overwhelming. Sometimes, the tools designed to streamline our lives leave us feeling tethered to screens, over-stimulated, and disconnected from the real world.

That's where the idea of a **tech detox** comes in. In a world of constant notifications, scrolling, and reliance on AI for even the smallest tasks, it's easy to feel like we're "always on." Taking a step back to reset isn't just refreshing—it's vital for our well-being.

Finding Balance with Digital Wellness

Digital wellness isn't about abandoning technology altogether; it's about using it intentionally to enhance your life without letting it consume your time or energy. Here are some strategies to find that balance:

- **Set Tech-Free Boundaries**
- Create designated times or spaces where screens are off-limits. For example, declare your dining table a phone-free zone or commit to winding down in the evening without checking emails or social media. My favorite? The "bedroom ban"—no phones, tablets, or laptops allowed. It's a simple rule that has transformed my sleep and my evenings.
- **Take Screen-Free Breaks**
- Ever find yourself aimlessly scrolling, only to realize an hour has disappeared? Scheduling intentional breaks from technology can help. Whether it's taking a walk, reading a physical book, or simply enjoying a cup of coffee without your phone, these moments of mindfulness can recharge your mental battery. Personally, I find that stepping outside for a quick nature walk or playing an old board game with my kids works wonders.
- **Use Technology with Purpose**
- Remember, you're still the one in charge. AI can organize your schedule, refine your skincare routine, or even give you a pep talk on tough days—but you decide how it fits into your life. Whether it's suggesting workout routines, recommending products, or generating social media ideas, **you hold the power**. Use AI as a tool to enhance your life, not run it.

Digital Detox Retreats: A Reset for the Mind and Body

For those feeling particularly overwhelmed, a **digital detox retreat** can be a game-changer. Imagine spending a weekend in nature, practicing mindfulness, and completely unplugging from your devices. No notifications, no emails, no distractions —just time to reconnect with yourself and the people around you.

These retreats are gaining popularity as more people seek to reset their relationship with technology. Even if you can't get away for a full retreat, dedicating a day or a weekend at home to being screen-free can be incredibly restorative. Use the time to journal, practice yoga, or simply enjoy the quiet. It's amazing how much mental clarity you can gain when the digital noise is turned off.

THE BOTTOM LINE

AI and technology are incredible tools that can make our lives easier, more efficient, and even more enjoyable. But like any tool, they need to be used mindfully. By setting boundaries, taking intentional breaks, and embracing the occasional tech detox, we can strike a balance that allows us to benefit from technology while staying grounded in the present. After all, the ultimate control lies in your hands—AI is here to support, not replace, your decisions.

CONCLUSION: EMPOWERING WOMEN WITH AI AND BALANCE

Artificial intelligence is no longer just a futuristic buzzword— it's a tool that's revolutionizing how we approach beauty, wellness, and everyday life. From personalized skincare routines to planning family adventures with ease, AI empowers us to live smarter, healthier, and more balanced lives. It's like having a personal assistant, wellness coach, and beauty expert rolled into one, helping to lighten the mental load that so many women carry daily.

However, as much as AI can enhance our lives, it's essential to stay mindful of balance. Technology should serve as a tool to simplify, not a crutch that leads to overwhelm. Creating intentional boundaries—whether through tech-free family dinners, mindful breaks, or moments of self-care without screens—is just as critical as leveraging AI to optimize our routines. These moments of stillness and connection are where true beauty and well-being are cultivated.

The beauty of AI lies in its ability to personalize and stream-line, but the power to create a fulfilling life ultimately rests in your hands. AI is your partner in the journey, offering insights and solutions that align with your needs, but it's you who decides how to use these tools. By blending the convenience of technology with mindfulness, you can enjoy the best of both worlds.

So, let AI inspire you to glow, grow, and thrive. Embrace its innovations to ease your day-to-day, but don't forget to step back and savor the present. Balance is where the magic happens, and when you pair AI's cutting-edge capabilities with mindful living, you create a life that is not only smarter but also more joyful and fulfilling.

This is the essence of modern beauty and wellness—harnessing innovation without losing sight of what makes life meaningful: connection, self-care, and living in the moment.

CHAPTER 20
HORMONAL HEALTH AND BEAUTY
MASTERING THE ART OF BALANCE THROUGH BIOHACKING

Let's be honest—our hormones have a way of keeping us on our toes. One moment, we're glowing with confidence, and the next, we're battling breakouts, fatigue, or a sudden bad hair day. From puberty to menopause (and all the stages in between), hormones shape so much more than just our mood. They influence how we look, feel, and function every single day.

But here's the empowering part: understanding your hormonal health doesn't have to feel like an uphill battle. By learning to recognize your body's natural rhythms and leveraging the power of **biohacking**, you can create harmony between your hormones and your beauty routine. Imagine having more good skin days, better energy, and a deeper sense of balance—all by working *with* your body rather than against it.

This chapter is all about giving you the tools and knowledge to do just that. Whether you're curious about syncing your skincare routine with your menstrual cycle, boosting your hair health during hormonal shifts, or simply reclaiming control over your body, you're in the right place. Hormonal health isn't just science—it's an art, and together, we'll unlock the secrets to mastering it.

Let's dive in and discover how to thrive through every hormonal twist and turn life throws our way. Because when you're in sync with your body, true beauty shines from the inside out.

HOW HORMONAL FLUCTUATIONS AFFECT YOUR SKIN, HAIR, AND MOOD

Hormones like estrogen, progesterone, and testosterone play key roles in regulating not only your reproductive system but also your beauty. Let's break down how these hormonal shifts can show up on your skin, hair, and even your mood.

- **Skin:** Ever notice how your skin seems to have a mind of its own, sometimes glowing and flawless, and other times breaking out like you're back in high school? That's your hormones at work. Estrogen, for instance, helps your skin stay plump and hydrated, while progesterone can sometimes lead to excess oil production, which triggers breakouts. And don't even get me started on **testosterone**—although it's usually in smaller amounts in women, when it spikes, it can definitely cause unwanted acne.

I've even had a few friends who, despite using the best skincare products and sticking to a strict routine, still struggled with **melasma** or **skin discoloration** on their faces. No matter how careful they were, those dark patches would show up, and it wasn't until later that they realized it was their **hormones** playing tricks on them. It's frustrating because you feel like you're doing everything right, but hormones can be a wild card that's hard to control.

So, what's really going on here? The science behind this is linked to how **estrogen** and **progesterone** interact with **melanocytes**, the cells responsible for producing **melanin**. When **estrogen levels rise**—as they do during pregnancy or when taking hormonal birth control—these hormones can stimulate melanocytes to produce more melanin, which can lead to **hyperpigmentation,** such as melasma.

What makes this even worse is that **sun exposure** acts as a major trigger. When your skin is exposed to UV rays, the combination of increased estrogen and sunlight can cause your melanocytes to go into overdrive, producing even more melanin. This is why women often notice that their melasma or skin discoloration worsens during **pregnancy** (also known as the "pregnancy mask") or when they're on **hormonal birth control**, as these factors cause a surge in estrogen, which, when combined with sun exposure, can lead to more pronounced pigmentation.

So, while hormonal fluctuations and skin discoloration may be **unpredictable**, you can still take steps to manage their effects. It's all about understanding the underlying causes and knowing that sometimes, even the best skincare routine isn't enough to counteract what's happening beneath the surface.

Here's what you can do to manage the effects:

1. **Sun Protection**: Wear a **broad-spectrum sunscreen** with at least **SPF 30** every single day, even when it's cloudy or you're indoors. Reapply every two hours if you're spending time outside, and consider wearing protective clothing like hats or sunglasses. Sun exposure is a major trigger, so this step is crucial.
2. **Topical Treatments**: Products like **hydroquinone** (which reduces melanin production), **retinoids** (which boost cell turnover), **azelaic acid** (for anti-inflammatory benefits), and **vitamin C** (for brightening) can help reduce the appearance of dark spots over time.
3. **Consider Hormonal Alternatives**: If you're on **hormonal birth control** and find your melasma worsening, speak with your doctor about switching to a non-hormonal contraceptive method. Reducing the impact of estrogen could make a difference.

4. **In-Office Treatments**: Professional options like **chemical peels** and **laser therapy** can help reduce discoloration, but these should be done under the guidance of a dermatologist, as improper use of lasers on melasma can worsen the condition.
5. **Lifestyle Adjustments**: Stress can affect your hormones, and managing stress through **yoga**, **meditation**, or **exercise** can help keep your hormones in balance, which may improve your skin. A balanced diet with plenty of antioxidants and healthy fats can also support your skin health.
6. **Consistency**: Managing melasma takes time, so be patient. Consistency with sun protection and skincare treatments is key, as results can take months to show.

By following these steps, you can minimize the impact of hormonal fluctuations on your skin. While you may not be able to control your hormones entirely, these strategies will help you manage their effects and keep your skin looking its best.

MOOD AND HORMONES: UNDERSTANDING THE ROLLERCOASTER

Let's talk about the elephant in the room: hormones. They can be our best friends one moment and our toughest critics the next. If you've ever wondered why you feel on top of the world one week and then tear up watching a rerun of a cat food commercial the next, you're not alone. Hormones play a massive role in shaping our mood, energy levels, and emotional balance, and understanding their influence can make the ups and downs a little easier to navigate.

The Luteal Phase: The "Pre-Period" Zone

The luteal phase, which occurs in the week or so before your period, is like nature's emotional boot camp. This phase starts after ovulation, and it's when the hormone progesterone takes center stage. Progesterone is often called the "calming hormone" because it can promote feelings of relaxation and help with sleep. But let's be real: instead of feeling serene, this phase often leaves us tired, cranky, and searching for chocolate.

Why? Well, while progesterone tries to keep things calm, it also slows everything down. Your metabolism shifts, your energy can dip, and your body starts preparing for either a pregnancy or your next cycle. Add in the fact that estrogen, the "feel-good hormone," drops during this phase, and you have a recipe for mood swings, irritability, and even anxiety.

Why Do We Feel So Emotional?

When estrogen levels drop and progesterone increases, it creates a hormonal imbalance that can affect neurotransmitters like serotonin—the brain chemical responsible for happiness and emotional regulation. This imbalance can make you feel:

- **Irritable:** Small things that usually wouldn't bother you might feel like a big deal. (Hello, "why didn't you put your socks in the laundry basket?" fights.)
- **Anxious:** A racing mind or an unsettled feeling can creep in, even without a clear reason.
- **Tired:** Your body's slower pace can make you feel like you're wading through molasses.
- **Down:** That drop in serotonin can leave you feeling blue, even if nothing's wrong.

How to Support Your Mood During the Luteal Phase

The good news is that you can take simple steps to support your mood and energy during this time. It's all about understanding what your body needs and being kind to yourself.

1. Nourish with the Right Foods:

- Magnesium-rich foods like dark chocolate (yes, really!), nuts, and spinach can help stabilize mood and reduce cramps.

- Omega-3 fatty acids from salmon, walnuts, or chia seeds are great for supporting brain health and reducing inflammation.
- Complex carbs like oats, quinoa, or sweet potatoes can boost serotonin levels naturally.

2. Move Your Body (Even When You Don't Want To):

- Gentle exercises like yoga, walking, or stretching can release endorphins—the body's natural mood boosters.
- If you're up for it, a quick dance session in your living room can do wonders for lifting your spirits.

3. Prioritize Rest and Sleep:

- Progesterone makes you feel sleepy for a reason—your body is asking for rest. Listen to it.
- Create a calming nighttime routine with herbal teas, a warm bath, or some light reading.

4. Herbal Helpers:

- Chasteberry (Vitex): Known for balancing hormones and alleviating PMS symptoms.
- Ashwagandha: An adaptogen that helps the body manage stress and reduce anxiety.

5. Stay Connected:

- Talk to friends, share your feelings, or vent if needed. Sometimes, just knowing you're not alone can make a world of difference.

A GENTLE REMINDER

If you find yourself snapping at loved ones or feeling over-whelmed during this phase, remember: you're not "overreacting." You're human. Hormonal fluctuations are a normal part of life, and they don't define who you are. Instead of fighting your body, work with it. Take the luteal phase as a reminder to slow down, practice self-care, and treat yourself with the compassion you deserve.

THE TAKEAWAY

Hormones may have a mind of their own, but you can regain control by tuning into what your body needs. By supporting your mood through nourishing foods, gentle movement, and rest, you'll navigate the luteal phase with a little more ease. And when all else fails? Remember: this too shall pass—and there's always chocolate.

MENSTRUAL SYNCING WITH YOUR WELLNESS ROUTINE

Instead of fighting your hormones, why not work with them? Menstrual syncing is all about aligning your wellness and beauty routines with the natural phases of your cycle. It may sound fancy, but it's pretty straightforward once you get the hang of it. And trust me, it makes a world of difference.

By understanding the changes your body goes through each month, you can adjust your self-care, workouts, and skincare routines to better suit your needs. Let's break it down:

Phase 1: Follicular Phase (Days 1–14)

This phase starts on the first day of your period and lasts until ovulation. Estrogen levels gradually rise, which means more energy and glowing skin. Your body is in "prep mode," building the follicle that will release an egg.

What Happens:

- Energy and motivation increase.
- Skin looks brighter and more hydrated.

Wellness Syncing:

- **Skincare:** Gentle exfoliation and hydration can enhance your natural glow. Think light serums with hyaluronic acid and a soothing moisturizer to lock in hydration.
- **Exercise:** This is the time for high-energy workouts like cardio, strength training, or a fun dance class. You're likely feeling strong and capable, so make the most of it.
- **Mindset:** Use this productive, energetic phase to set goals, try something new, or tackle a challenging project.

Phase 2: Ovulation (Around Day 14)

Ovulation is when estrogen peaks, and your body is at its most fertile. This is your "power phase," with optimal blood flow, glowing skin, and heightened confidence. However, a slight increase in testosterone can also lead to subtle breakouts.

What Happens:

- Skin glows but may be prone to breakouts due to increased sebum production.
- You feel more confident and social.

Wellness Syncing:

- **Skincare:** Stick to your regular routine, but add spot treatments with ingredients like salicylic acid if you notice breakouts.
- **Exercise:** You're at peak energy—perfect for pushing your limits in workouts or trying something adventurous.
- **Lifestyle:** This is a great time for networking,

socializing, or scheduling important events. Your natural confidence is shining through.

Phase 3: Luteal Phase (Days 15–28)

As progesterone rises after ovulation, your body begins preparing for a potential pregnancy. This phase can bring fatigue, bloating, mood swings, and even oily skin or acne.

What Happens:

- Progesterone slows your metabolic processes, leading to tiredness and bloating.
- Mood swings occur as progesterone impacts serotonin levels.
- Skin may become oily or breakout prone.
- Why These Symptoms Occur:
- Fatigue: Progesterone has a sedative effect, which helps your body conserve energy.
- Mood Swings: Fluctuations in serotonin can trigger irritability, sadness, or anxiety.
- Bloating: Progesterone relaxes digestive muscles, slowing digestion and causing water retention.

Wellness Syncing:

- **Skincare:** Focus on calming, anti-inflammatory products like niacinamide or green tea extract to control oil and soothe skin.
- **Exercise:** Switch to restorative workouts like yoga, walking, or light stretching. Your body will thank you for the gentler pace.
- **Self-Care:** Prioritize stress-reducing practices like meditation, deep breathing, or warm baths.

Phase 4: Menstruation (Days 1–5 of the New Cycle)

When estrogen and progesterone drop, you may feel tired and notice duller skin. This is your body's time to reset and release what it no longer needs.

What Happens:

- Energy levels are at their lowest.
- Skin can appear dry or lackluster.

Wellness Syncing:

- **Skincare:** Hydrate, hydrate, hydrate! Use nourishing oils or moisturizers to combat dryness and restore your glow.
- **Exercise:** Give yourself permission to rest. If you do exercise, opt for gentle activities like restorative yoga or a calming walk.
- **Mindset:** Embrace this phase as a time for reflection and rest. Journaling or mindful activities can help you recharge mentally.

PREVENTING THE NEGATIVE EFFECTS OF HORMONAL CHANGES

While we can't completely control our hormones, we can minimize their impact by making smart lifestyle choices:

1. Balance Your Diet:

- Incorporate omega-3 fatty acids (from salmon and walnuts) and leafy greens to reduce inflammation.
- Limit sugar and refined carbs, which can worsen mood swings and hormonal imbalances.

2. Smart Supplements:

- Magnesium: Helps with cramps, fatigue, and mood stabilization.
- Vitamin D: Supports serotonin production and overall hormonal health.
- Evening Primrose Oil: Known to ease PMS symptoms and improve skin health.

3. Exercise Wisely:

- Match your workouts to your cycle. For example, go hard during the follicular and ovulation phases, and take it easy during the luteal and menstrual phases. This not only helps regulate hormones but also prevents burnout.

4. Hydration:

- Drink plenty of water throughout your cycle. Dehydration can exacerbate bloating, cramps, and mood swings.

THE BEAUTY OF MENSTRUAL SYNCING

By syncing your wellness routine with your menstrual cycle, you're not just reacting to hormonal changes—you're working with them. This approach allows you to embrace your body's natural rhythms, optimize your energy, and balance your beauty and wellness routines.

Remember, your cycle isn't a burden; it's a powerful guide that helps you connect with your body and take care of yourself in ways that feel intuitive and nourishing. So, listen to your body, honor its needs, and thrive in every phase!

BIOHACKING FOR HORMONAL HEALTH: A MODERN WELLNESS UPGRADE

Let's be honest: managing hormones can sometimes feel like trying to wrangle a herd of cats. They're unpredictable, moody, and occasionally leave you wondering, "Is it just me, or is my body plotting against me?" Enter biohacking—a fancy term for simple, science-backed strategies that help you work with your body instead of fighting it. Think of it as your personal toolkit for optimizing wellness, beauty, and balance.

Cold Showers: A Refreshing Reset for Your Hormones

The idea of stepping into an icy shower might sound more like a punishment than a perk, but hear me out. Cold showers offer some surprisingly powerful benefits for your mood, skin, and hormonal balance. It's like a mini wake-up call for your entire system!

How It Works: When cold water hits your skin, it causes your blood vessels to constrict (hello, goosebumps!). This redirects blood flow to your core, improving circulation. Once you're out of the cold, your vessels dilate, boosting oxygen and nutrient delivery to your skin and organs.

Hormonal Boosts:

- **Stress Relief:** Cold exposure triggers a release of endorphins and norepinephrine, giving you a natural high and reducing cortisol (the stress hormone). Who doesn't need a little less stress?
- **Energy Lift:** Cold showers activate your mitochondria—your body's power plants—giving you more energy to tackle the day (or at least that mountain of laundry).
- **How to Start:** If plunging into an ice-cold shower sounds like torture, start small. End your usual warm shower with 15–30 seconds of cold water. Gradually increase the duration as you get used to it. It's a quick,

no-cost way to feel rejuvenated, even if it's just your secret weapon for groggy mornings.

Infrared Saunas: Sweat It Out, Glow It Up

Imagine lying in a cozy warmth that not only relaxes you but also detoxifies your body and improves your skin. That's the magic of infrared saunas. Unlike traditional saunas that heat the air, infrared saunas use light waves to gently warm your body from within, offering deeper health benefits.

Why They're Amazing:

- **Detox Support:** Infrared heat helps you sweat out toxins, including those pesky endocrine disruptors that can mess with your hormones.
- **Stress Reduction:** It's like a warm hug for your nervous system, helping to lower cortisol and leave you feeling calm and centered.
- **Skin Love:** Increased blood flow promotes collagen production, giving your skin that post-sauna glow.
- **How to Use:** Aim for 20–30 minutes, 2–3 times a week. Remember to hydrate before and after to replenish what you've lost through sweat. Think of it as self-care with a scientific twist—your hormones (and skin!) will thank you.

Herbal Therapy: Nature's Hormonal Whisperers

When it comes to hormonal balance, Mother Nature has your back. Adaptogens, like ashwagandha and maca, are herbs that help your body adapt to stress and find equilibrium. They're like that calm, supportive friend who always knows just what to say.

Why It Works:

- **Ashwagandha:** Known as the "queen of calm," this Ayurvedic herb supports your adrenal glands, helping to regulate cortisol levels and promote restful sleep. It's perfect for managing those chaotic hormonal shifts that leave you feeling frazzled.

- **Maca:** A Peruvian powerhouse, maca nourishes your endocrine system, balancing estrogen and progesterone. It's particularly helpful for PMS symptoms, menopausal hot flashes, and even boosting libido. Yes, please!

Science Says:

- Studies show that ashwagandha can reduce cortisol levels by up to 30%, easing anxiety and fatigue.
- Maca has been linked to improved mood, hormonal balance, and energy levels by regulating the hypothalamic-pituitary-adrenal (HPA) axis.

How to Incorporate:

- Add maca powder to your smoothies or oatmeal for a nutty, caramel-like flavor that's as delicious as it is beneficial.
- Enjoy a calming cup of ashwagandha tea in the evening—it's like a bedtime story for your hormones.

IS BIOHACKING RIGHT FOR YOU?

Biohacking isn't about perfection or doing it all at once. It's about experimenting with small, intentional changes that make your life easier, your energy more consistent, and your skin a little glowier. Whether it's tracking your cycle, embracing the chill of a cold shower, or trying an adaptogenic herb, the key is to find what works for you.

Start small, stay curious, and don't be afraid to tweak your routine. After all, your hormones aren't the boss of you—you're the boss of them. Now, go ahead and biohack your way to balance, beauty, and brilliance!

CONCLUSION: EMPOWERING YOUR HORMONAL HEALTH JOURNEY

Your hormonal health is more than just a collection of cycles and symptoms—it's a reflection of your body's inner harmony and resilience. Understanding and embracing the ebb and flow of your hormones isn't about controlling every fluctuation but about creating balance and synergy. This chapter isn't just a guide—it's an invitation to reclaim your wellness with purpose, curiosity, and self-love.

By syncing your wellness routine with your natural rhythms, you're not only enhancing your beauty and vitality but also cultivating a deeper connection with your body. Whether it's through tracking your cycle, nourishing yourself with adaptogenic herbs, or exploring the invigorating power of cold showers and infrared saunas, every small step you take builds a foundation of self-care that supports you through every phase of life.

Remember, your hormones aren't the enemy—they're a powerful ally when understood and nurtured. Lean into the wisdom of your body, embrace the tools of modern biohacking, and let your journey inspire others to do the same. Aging gracefully, thriving vibrantly, and living authentically—it all starts with honoring your hormones and celebrating the amazing woman you are.

Now is the time to step into your power. Your body, mind, and spirit are worth every moment of care you give them. Let this chapter be the beginning of a beautiful partnership with yourself—a relationship rooted in strength, wisdom, and grace. Your best self is always within reach; all you need to do is listen, nurture, and shine.

CHAPTER 21

HOLISTIC WELLNESS AND BREAST CANCER

A JOURNEY OF STRENGTH, HEALING, AND EMPOWERMENT

A MESSAGE OF CARE AND AWARENESS

Breast cancer is a deeply personal and emotional topic for me. As a nurse, I once held the hand of a young female patient as she took her final breath, leaving behind a grieving husband and young children. The pain and heartbreak of that moment will stay with me forever. It was a powerful reminder of how precious life is and how important it is to take steps to protect our health.

This experience is why I feel compelled to include this chapter. My hope is to share knowledge and tools that can empower women to take charge of their health. This chapter is not just about breast cancer; it's about embracing a holistic approach to prevention, creating a lifestyle rooted in balance and wellness, and fostering habits that can make a difference. Together, we'll explore actionable steps to reduce risk, prioritize early detection, and live with resilience and hope. Let's turn awareness into action—for ourselves, for those we love, and for the futures we want to protect.

SECTION 1: PREVENTION THROUGH HOLISTIC LIVING

Cancer prevention isn't just about big, sweeping changes—it's about small, intentional choices that add up to big impacts at the cellular level. Every bite we take, every step we walk, and every moment we spend prioritizing our well-being is a step toward protecting ourselves. Let me share some science-backed ways to nourish your body and lower your risk of breast cancer—practices I've come to embrace after witnessing how powerful prevention can be.

1. Nourish Your Body with Cancer-Fighting Foods

Food as Medicine isn't just a buzzword; it's a reality. The right foods don't just fill your belly—they actively help your cells repair, defend, and thrive.

Cruciferous Vegetables: Broccoli, Kale, Cauliflower, Brussels Sprouts

- **Why They Work:** These veggies are packed with sulforaphane and indole-3-carbinol, nature's detox agents. They help flush out harmful substances and may even stop tumors in their tracks.
- **What They Do in Cells:** Sulforaphane can "turn on" your body's natural defense system, activating enzymes that neutralize carcinogens. It even nudges rogue cancer cells toward self-destruction (talk about tough love!).
- **How to Add Them:** Roast broccoli for dinner, toss kale in your smoothie, or sauté Brussels sprouts with garlic—it's not just healthy, it's delicious.

Antioxidant-Rich Foods: Berries, Spinach, Tomatoes

- **Why They Work:** Antioxidants are like little bodyguards for your cells, neutralizing free radicals that can damage DNA and kickstart cancer.

- **What They Do in Cells:** By stabilizing these harmful molecules, antioxidants prevent them from wreaking havoc. Think of them as your cellular cleanup crew, ensuring everything runs smoothly.
- **How to Add Them:** Snack on blueberries, whip up a spinach salad, or enjoy a bowl of tomato soup. Easy, right?

Healthy Fats: Avocados, Walnuts, Flaxseeds

- **Why They Work:** Omega-3 fatty acids fight inflammation, a major player in cancer development. Chronic inflammation can damage cells, but healthy fats step in to calm things down.
- **What They Do in Cells:** Omega-3s act like diplomats, reducing the chaos of inflammation and even slowing tumor growth.
- **How to Add Them:** Add a few slices of avocado to your toast, sprinkle walnuts on your oatmeal, or blend flaxseeds into your smoothie.

Green Tea: The Anti-Cancer Brew

- **Why It Works:** Packed with catechins like EGCG, green tea is a cellular superhero. It blocks cancer cells from multiplying and cuts off their blood supply.
- **What It Does in Cells:** Catechins disrupt cancer cell growth and boost your body's natural detox system.
- **How to Add It:** Sip a cup of green tea in the morning or afternoon—it's a habit worth brewing.

2. Limit Red Meat and Sugar

I get it—burgers and sweets are tempting, but they might not be worth the risk.

Red Meat:

- **The Concern:** Overcooked red meat releases harmful chemicals (HCAs and PAHs) that can damage DNA. Plus, the heme iron in red meat can cause oxidative stress in your gut.
- **What Happens in Cells:** These harmful compounds can lead to mutations, increasing cancer risk.

Sugar:

- **The Concern:** Cancer cells love sugar. A diet high in sugar can lead to insulin resistance and fuel cancer growth.
- **What Happens in Cells:** High insulin levels trigger cell proliferation, creating a favorable environment for cancer.
- **How to Cut Back:** Swap soda for water, choose whole fruits over desserts, and gradually reduce processed snacks.

3. Stay Active: Movement as Medicine

Exercise doesn't just tone your body—it strengthens your cells.

- **Why It Works:** Physical activity reduces estrogen and insulin levels, two hormones that can fuel certain cancers. It also boosts immune surveillance, helping your body spot and destroy abnormal cells.
- **What It Does in Cells:** Exercise lowers inflammation, improves DNA repair, and keeps your metabolism humming.
- **How to Add It:** Start with 30 minutes of brisk walking, yoga, or strength training a few times a week. Bonus points if you get outside and soak up some vitamin D!

4. Mind Your Environment: Reduce Toxic Exposures

Everyday products can hide harmful chemicals, but with a few swaps, you can minimize exposure.

- **Natural Cleaning Products:** Choose ones free from parabens and phthalates, which can disrupt hormones and increase cancer risk.
- **Plastic-Free Living:** Switch to glass or stainless steel to avoid BPA, a chemical linked to hormone-sensitive cancers.

The Power of Holistic Choices

Here's the takeaway: prevention starts with daily habits. The foods you eat, the steps you take, and the products you use all contribute to your body's ability to protect itself. It's not about overhauling your life overnight—it's about making small, meaningful changes that add up over time.

Because here's the truth: your body is on your side. With the right care, you can create an environment where your cells thrive, inflammation stays in check, and cancer stands no chance.

Now, let's get started—one step, one meal, and one choice at a time. And hey, don't forget to savor that green tea!

SECTION 2: EARLY DETECTION IS EMPOWERMENT

When it comes to breast cancer, early detection isn't just a strategy—it's a lifesaver. The earlier you spot potential signs, the better your chances of effective treatment and recovery. Think of this as tuning in to your body's whispers before they become shouts.

1. Monthly Self-Exams

Performing monthly breast self-exams is like checking in with an old friend—familiarity matters. Spend a few minutes every month getting to know your breasts.

- **What to Look For:** Changes in size, shape, texture, or any unusual lumps. Notice any dimpling, redness, or discharge.
- **Why It's Important:** You are your body's best advocate. By knowing what's normal for you, you'll quickly spot anything that's not.
- **How to Do It:** Perform the exam a few days after your period ends, when your breasts are least likely to be swollen. Use the pads of your fingers in a circular motion, covering the entire breast and armpit area.

2. Routine Screenings

Regular screenings are non-negotiable when it comes to early detection.

- **Mammograms:** Women over 40 should have yearly mammograms or as recommended by their doctor. If you have a family history of breast cancer, talk to your healthcare provider about starting earlier.
- **Why It's Critical:** Mammograms can detect changes that are too small to feel, catching potential issues at their earliest, most treatable stages.
- **Pro Tip:** Mark it on your calendar or pair it with another annual event (like your birthday) to make it a consistent part of your routine.

3. Listen to Your Body

Your body has a way of sending signals when something's off—don't ignore them.

- **What to Watch For:** Unexplained fatigue, persistent pain, swelling, or changes in the breast tissue.
- **Why It Matters:** These symptoms don't always mean cancer, but addressing them early ensures peace of mind and timely action.
- **Remember:** Trust your intuition. If something feels wrong, seek medical advice promptly.

SECTION 3: UNDERSTANDING TREATMENTS FOR DIFFERENT STAGES OF BREAST CANCER

When it comes to breast cancer, the treatment path can feel overwhelming, especially when faced with medical jargon and tough decisions. But here's the thing: knowledge is empowering. By understanding the different treatments, you can approach your journey—or support someone else's—with confidence and clarity. Let's break it down together in a way that's less intimidating and more like a supportive chat over coffee.

Stage 0 and Early-Stage Breast Cancer (Stage I & II)

At this stage, the focus is on catching it early and stopping it in its tracks.

- **What to Expect:**
  - **Surgery:** Whether it's a lumpectomy (removing just the tumor) or a mastectomy (removing the entire breast), the goal is to eliminate cancer cells.
  - **Radiation Therapy:** Often, this comes after surgery to zap any lingering troublemakers.
  - **Hormone Therapy:** For hormone-sensitive cancers, doctors may use this to block or reduce estrogen, which can act like fuel for some tumors.
- **What It Feels Like:** Surgery and radiation focus on the area where cancer was found, so the side effects are generally localized—think soreness, skin changes, or fatigue. Hormone therapy, however, can shake

things up with hot flashes, mood swings, and even bone thinning. (Yes, it's a lot, but we'll get through this together.)

Locally Advanced Breast Cancer (Stage III)

When cancer is more advanced, treatments often involve a combination of strategies to achieve the best possible outcome.

- **What to Expect:**
  - **Chemotherapy:** Sometimes it's used before surgery (to shrink the tumor) or after (to clean up any stragglers).
  - **Targeted Therapy:** These fancy drugs go straight for specific proteins that help cancer cells grow, like HER2 inhibitors.
  - **Radiation Therapy:** Still part of the game plan for some cases.
- **What It Feels Like:** This is where chemo enters the chat—and it's known for being tough. Hair loss, nausea, and fatigue can make it feel like your body is waging a war (because it is). Targeted therapies are a bit kinder but still come with their own quirks, like fatigue or even heart-related side effects. Radiation can cause localized fatigue and skin irritation but is generally easier than chemo.

Side Effects of Chemotherapy: Why does it cause Heart-Related Issues?

Chemotherapy is a powerful tool in the fight against cancer, but it doesn't come without its challenges. While hair loss, nausea, and fatigue are the side effects most people associate with chemo, there's a lesser-known but significant concern: heart-related side effects.

Chemotherapy, particularly certain drugs like anthracyclines (e.g., doxorubicin) or HER2-targeted therapies (e.g., trastuzumab), can potentially harm the heart. These drugs can weaken the heart muscle, leading to a condition known as cardiotoxicity, which may result in symptoms like shortness of breath, swelling, or even congestive heart failure in severe cases. Other heart-related side effects include irregular heart rhythms (arrhythmias) and elevated blood pressure.

Why Does This Happen?

Chemotherapy works by targeting rapidly dividing cells, which is great for killing cancer cells. However, this mechanism can also inadvertently harm healthy cells, including those in the heart. Additionally, certain drugs can cause inflammation or damage to the lining of blood vessels, leading to cardiovascular issues over time.

What Can Be Done?

- **Baseline Heart Checks:** Before starting treatment, oncologists often recommend echocardiograms or other heart-function tests to establish a baseline.
- **Ongoing Monitoring:** Regular checkups can detect early signs of heart damage.
- **Heart-Protective Strategies:** Some medications, like dexrazoxane, can be used to protect the heart during chemotherapy. Additionally, lifestyle changes like regular exercise and a heart-healthy diet can provide added support.
- **Personalized Treatment Plans:** Adjusting chemotherapy doses or switching to less cardiotoxic drugs can minimize risk.

While the risk of heart-related side effects is real, proactive monitoring and intervention can help mitigate these effects, allowing patients to focus on their cancer treatment journey with greater peace of mind.

Metastatic Breast Cancer (Stage IV): Living with Advanced Disease

When breast cancer progresses to Stage IV, it means the cancer has spread beyond the breast and nearby lymph nodes to other parts of the body, such as the bones, liver, lungs, or brain. At this stage, the goal of treatment shifts from curing the disease to slowing its progression, managing symptoms, and enhancing quality of life.

What to Expect from Treatment

1. Chemotherapy and Targeted Therapy

- **What It Does:** Chemotherapy destroys cancer cells throughout the body, while targeted therapies like HER2 inhibitors specifically attack cancer cells with certain genetic markers.
- **How It Feels**: Chemotherapy side effects can include fatigue, nausea, and hair loss, while targeted therapies may lead to fewer systemic side effects but can still cause fatigue or heart-related issues.

2. Hormone Therapy

- **What It Does:** For hormone-receptor-positive breast cancer, hormone therapy blocks or reduces the effects of estrogen, which fuels cancer growth.
- **How It Feels:** Generally well-tolerated but may cause menopausal-like symptoms such as hot flashes, mood swings, and bone thinning.

3. Immunotherapy

- **What It Does:** This cutting-edge treatment boosts the immune system's ability to recognize and destroy cancer cells. Drugs like immune checkpoint inhibitors are making strides in treating certain types of breast cancer.

- **How It Feels:** Compared to chemotherapy, immunotherapy tends to be gentler, though it can still cause fatigue, skin rashes, or flu-like symptoms.

4. Palliative Care

- **What It Does:** This is an integral part of managing Stage IV cancer, focusing on symptom control, emotional support, and overall quality of life.
- **How It Feels:** Think of palliative care as your wellness team—helping you manage pain, cope with treatment side effects, and prioritize your comfort and well-being.

What It Feels Like: Navigating the Emotional and Physical Journey

Living with metastatic breast cancer is a marathon, not a sprint. Treatments are often ongoing, and side effects can accumulate over time. Fatigue is a common challenge, but staying connected to your healthcare team and exploring strategies like light exercise, nutrition, and mindfulness can help.

The silver lining? Treatments like immunotherapy are often less physically taxing, and the focus on palliative care ensures that your journey is centered on what matters most to you—your comfort, goals, and overall quality of life. Every step of the way, you're in control of your story, supported by a team dedicated to helping you live fully, even with the challenges of metastatic cancer.

Empowering Yourself Through Knowledge and Support

Living with metastatic breast cancer requires strength, adaptability, and a network of support. By understanding your treatment options, side effects, and available resources, you can actively participate in decisions about your care. Treatments continue to evolve, offering new hope and possibilities for improved quality of life. And through it all, remember: you are more than your diagnosis.

Which Treatment Hits the Hardest?

Let's be real—chemo has a reputation, and for good reason. It's systemic, meaning it doesn't just target cancer but also healthy, fast-growing cells like those in your hair, gut, and immune system. That's why it's often considered the toughest on the body. It's like a full-scale war, and your body feels every battle.

Radiation, on the other hand, is more like a precision strike. While you might feel fatigue or notice skin changes in the treated area, it's generally less draining than chemotherapy. Hormone therapy tends to be gentler, but it comes with its quirks, like hot flashes, mood changes, or bone thinning over time.

No matter which treatment you're navigating, remember: understanding the challenges is the first step to overcoming them. And with the right support—whether it's a compassionate care team, lifestyle adjustments, or complementary therapies—you can find ways to manage side effects and keep moving forward.

Wrapping It Up: Why This Matters

It's not about scaring you—it's about preparing you. When you know what to expect, the fear of the unknown starts to lose its grip. Yes, each treatment comes with its own set of challenges, but being informed allows you to approach them with courage, confidence, and even a touch of grace.

This journey isn't one you walk alone. The right knowledge, support, and mindset can make all the difference. In the next section, we'll explore how to nurture your body, soothe your mind, and embrace holistic wellness during treatment. Because while the fight against cancer may be tough, there are countless ways to make the path a little lighter, a little kinder, and a lot more empowering. You've got this—we'll take it step by step.

SECTION 4: SUPPORTING WELLNESS DURING TREATMENT

Undergoing breast cancer treatment is an intensely personal journey—unique to every woman and every story. While medical treatments like chemotherapy, radiation, and surgery focus on combating the disease, incorporating holistic wellness practices can bring balance, comfort, and a sense of control back into your life.

These practices aren't just "nice-to-haves." They're powerful tools to support your physical recovery, maintain emotional resilience, and help you reconnect with your inner strength. Let's explore practical ways to care for your body, mind, and spirit during this challenging but transformative time.

Gentle Nutrition for Each Treatment Type

When navigating breast cancer treatment, proper nutrition becomes a crucial ally. Every treatment—whether chemotherapy, radiation, surgery, or immunotherapy—impacts the body differently. Adapting your diet to meet your body's unique needs can ease side effects, promote healing, and boost overall well-being. Let's explore how to tailor your nutrition to the challenges of each treatment type.

Why Nutrition Matters

Treatments can deplete energy, alter digestion, and strain your immune system. The right foods provide essential nutrients, reduce inflammation, and enhance your body's ability to heal and recover. Here's a treatment-specific guide to gentle nutrition:

For Chemotherapy: Supporting a Sensitive System

Challenges: Chemotherapy is tough on fast-growing cells, affecting the lining of your gut and causing nausea, loss of appetite, and mouth sores.

What to Do:

1. **Easy-to-Digest Foods**: Opt for gentle, nutrient-packed options like smoothies. A blend of spinach, bananas, almond butter, and a splash of plant-based milk provides energy and essential nutrients without straining your stomach.
2. **Bone Broth**: Packed with collagen, amino acids, and minerals, bone broth supports tissue repair and soothes inflammation. Sip it warm for a comforting, healing boost.
3. **Ginger Tea**: Ginger's anti-nausea properties can be a lifesaver. Sip on ginger tea or keep ginger candies handy for quick relief.
4. **Small, Frequent Meals**: If large meals feel daunting, snack on nutrient-dense foods like almonds, berries, or whole-grain crackers throughout the day.

For Radiation Therapy: Replenishing and Hydrating

Challenges: Radiation can cause fatigue, dehydration, and difficulty swallowing (especially when targeting the chest or throat).

What to Do:

1. **Hydration is Key**: Radiation increases water loss, so stay hydrated. Try infused water with cucumber, lemon, or mint for a refreshing twist that encourages you to drink more.
2. **Soft Foods**: If swallowing becomes difficult, choose easily consumed options like mashed sweet potatoes, oatmeal, yogurt, or blended soups.

3. **Antioxidant-Rich Choices**: Foods like blueberries, oranges, and spinach combat oxidative stress caused by radiation. Their vitamins and phytochemicals support cellular repair and reduce inflammation.

For Surgery: Fueling Recovery

Challenges: Surgery demands extra energy and nutrients for tissue repair, wound healing, and immune function.

What to Do:

1. **Protein Power**: Protein is your body's building block. Include lean meats, eggs, lentils, and tofu to accelerate tissue regeneration.
2. **Vitamin C Boost**: Vitamin C promotes collagen production, essential for wound healing. Snack on strawberries, oranges, and bell peppers to give your body what it needs.
3. **Zinc for Recovery**: Zinc plays a critical role in immune function and healing. Pumpkin seeds, chickpeas, and fortified cereals are excellent sources.

For Immunotherapy: Balancing Inflammation

Challenges: Immunotherapy enhances your immune response but can cause inflammation and fatigue as side effects.

What to Do:

1. **Anti-Inflammatory Diet**: Embrace foods like turmeric (with black pepper for absorption), fatty fish like salmon, and walnuts to reduce inflammation.
2. **Probiotics for Gut Health**: A healthy microbiome supports your immune system. Incorporate yogurt, kefir, or fermented foods like kimchi and sauerkraut into your meals.
3. **Energy-Boosting Snacks**: Fatigue can sneak up on

you, so keep energy levels stable with trail mix made of nuts, seeds, and dried fruit.

Extra Tips for Holistic Support

- **Listen to Your Body**: Cravings and aversions are common during treatment. Honor what feels good to eat while ensuring balanced nutrition.
- **Avoid Irritants**: Steer clear of spicy, overly acidic, or fried foods that can aggravate sensitive digestion.
- **Mindful Eating**: Chew slowly and eat in a calm environment to improve digestion and reduce stress on your system.

Why This Matters

The food on your plate is more than just sustenance; it's an active part of your healing process. Tailoring your nutrition to each treatment type allows you to better navigate side effects, recover faster, and feel empowered in your journey.

Remember, small, thoughtful choices in your diet can make a big difference—not just for your body but for your spirit. Whether it's sipping warm bone broth, savoring antioxidant-rich berries, or nourishing yourself with a creamy smoothie, these moments of care are acts of resilience and love for yourself.

MINDFULNESS AND RELAXATION: CALM THE MIND, HEAL THE BODY

Why It's Important

Cancer treatment is more than a physical challenge—it's a mental and emotional battlefield. The stress, uncertainty, and constant adjustments can feel overwhelming, but incorporating mindfulness and relaxation techniques can be a powerful way to reclaim control. These practices not only help you manage stress but also promote healing by reducing inflammation, improving sleep, and calming the nervous system. Let's turn your moments of chaos into pockets of calm, one mindful breath at a time.

For Chemotherapy: Finding Calm Amidst the Chaos

- **Guided Imagery:** Close your eyes and picture your body as a garden. Visualize each treatment as rain nourishing the soil, helping healthy cells grow stronger while washing away the weeds. Guided imagery has been shown to reduce stress and enhance a sense of healing during treatment.
- **Calming Music:** Create a playlist of soft instrumentals or nostalgic tunes that make you smile. Research shows that music can lower cortisol levels and reduce anxiety, making those long hours in the chemo chair feel a bit more bearable.
- **Actionable Tip:** Bring headphones or a portable speaker to chemo sessions to immerse yourself in music that soothes your soul. Pair it with deep breathing for double the calm.

For Radiation Therapy: Turning Tension Into Tranquility

- **Deep Breathing Exercises:** Use the 4-7-8 technique: inhale for 4 seconds, hold for 7, and exhale for 8. This simple practice activates the parasympathetic nervous system, helping your body relax before and during treatments.
- **Gratitude Journaling:** Even in difficult times, there's something to be thankful for. Write down three things you're grateful for each day. Gratitude can shift your focus from fear to positivity, improving mental resilience.
- **Actionable Tip:** Keep a small gratitude journal by

your bed and jot down thoughts before sleeping. It's a gentle way to end the day on a positive note.

For Surgery: Preparing and Recovering With Grace

- **Meditation for Recovery:** Apps like Calm, Insight Timer, or Headspace offer guided meditations specifically for stress relief and healing. These can ease pre-surgery jitters and promote relaxation post-op.
- **Progressive Muscle Relaxation:** Lie down comfortably and focus on tensing and releasing each muscle group, starting from your toes and working upward. This reduces pre-surgery anxiety and aids relaxation.
- **Actionable Tip:** Start meditating a week before surgery to build the habit. Post-surgery, use progressive relaxation to ease discomfort and reconnect with your body.

For Immunotherapy: Grounding Your Mind and Boosting Recovery

- **Nature Walks:** A short 10-minute stroll surrounded by greenery can reduce stress hormones, calm inflammation, and clear your mind. Nature truly is a healer.
- **Mantras for Strength:** Repeat empowering affirmations like, "I am strong, I am healing, I am resilient." Mantras help anchor your thoughts, turning self-doubt into self-belief.
- **Actionable Tip:** Create a dedicated "nature and mantra" routine—start your day with a brisk walk and close it with a calming affirmation session.

NATURAL SKINCARE FOR SENSITIVE SKIN

Why Skincare Matters

Cancer treatments, whether chemotherapy, radiation, or immunotherapy, can leave your skin feeling dry, sensitive, and irritated. Protecting and nourishing your skin is about more than appearance—it's about comfort and self-care during a difficult time. Here's how to care for your skin based on your treatment type.

For Chemotherapy: Soothing the Surface

- **Hydration Heroes:** Use fragrance-free, hypoallergenic moisturizers like Cetaphil or natural oils like coconut or jojoba. Apply them right after showering to lock in moisture.
- **Lip Love:** Dry, chapped lips are common. Keep an SPF lip balm on hand to hydrate and protect against sun exposure.
- **Actionable Tip:** Carry a small skincare kit to chemo sessions with a gentle moisturizer, lip balm, and hydrating mist for instant comfort.

For Radiation Therapy: Calming Redness and Irritation

- **Aloe Vera Gel:** Apply pure, chilled aloe vera to soothe burns and reduce redness. Its anti-inflammatory properties provide instant relief.
- **Breathable Fabrics:** Avoid harsh materials like polyester and stick to soft, natural fabrics like cotton to minimize friction on sensitive skin.
- **Actionable Tip:** Keep aloe vera gel in the fridge for a cooling effect and layer on loose cotton clothes to let your skin breathe.

For Surgery: Healing Skin, Healing Scars

- **Scar Therapy:** Once cleared by your doctor, use silicone gel sheets or vitamin E oil to minimize scarring and promote healing.
- **Stay Hydrated:** Skin heals faster when hydrated. Drink plenty of water and use hydrating skincare to support recovery from the inside out.
- **Actionable Tip:** Create a post-surgery skincare routine with scar treatments and hydrating serums to make recovery feel intentional and empowering.

For Immunotherapy: Managing Inflammation

- **Soothing Ingredients:** Look for products containing chamomile, calendula, or oat extract to calm irritation and inflammation.
- **Barrier Creams:** Protect compromised skin with gentle, fragrance-free barrier creams that lock in moisture and shield against irritants.
- **Actionable Tip:** Consult your oncologist or dermatologist for skin-safe product recommendations tailored to your needs.

FINAL THOUGHT

Mindfulness, relaxation, and skincare aren't just luxuries—they're vital tools to navigate the journey of cancer treatment. With a little effort and intentionality, these small acts of self-care can make a big difference in how you feel physically and emotionally. Remember, this is your journey, and every step you take toward comfort and healing is a step toward reclaiming your strength. You've got this!

WRAPPING IT UP: THE POWER OF RESILIENCE AND CONNECTION

Every woman's journey through cancer treatment is unique, but what binds us is our need for support, comfort, and empowerment. Holistic approaches like nourishing your body with healing foods, calming your mind with mindfulness, and finding strength in restorative practices are not just about surviving—they're about thriving. These strategies remind you of your inherent resilience and the beauty of life, even amid its challenges.

And let's not forget the power of community. Whether it's leaning on loved ones, joining a support group, or simply sharing your story, connection heals in ways that medicine cannot. Asking for help is not a sign of weakness—it's a testament to your strength and humanity.

SECTION 5: THRIVING AFTER RECOVERY

Emerging from breast cancer treatment is not just about healing physically; it's a transformative time of renewal, self-discovery, and growth. It's about reclaiming your body, mind, and spirit while embracing the lessons learned along the way. Let's explore how to step into this next chapter with grace, intention, and joy.

1. Rebuilding Strength: Rediscovering Your Body's Power

Your body has been through a lot, and recovery means rebuilding gently and mindfully.

- **Gentle Strength Training**: Start small with light weightlifting or resistance band exercises to regain muscle tone, improve bone density, and restore vitality. Celebrate small wins, like feeling stronger or steadier over time.

- **Walking Therapy**: There's something magical about putting one foot in front of the other. Walking is free, easy, and great for both physical and mental health.
- **Restorative Yoga**: This gentle, supportive practice is about healing through movement and stillness, calming your mind, and reconnecting with your body.

Restorative Yoga: Healing Through Movement and Stillness

Cancer treatments often leave the body feeling tense, depleted, and disconnected. Restorative yoga meets you where you are, offering poses that support physical recovery and emotional resilience.

Why Restorative Yoga?

Restorative yoga reduces physical discomfort, anxiety, and stress while gently nurturing your body's natural healing processes. It helps you feel present and empowered, turning moments of rest into acts of self-care.

Simple Poses to Try:

1. **Child's Pose (Balasana)**
   - Gently stretches the back, hips, and shoulders while calming the mind.
   - Sit back on your heels, stretch your arms forward, and rest your forehead on a pillow or the floor.
2. **Reclined Butterfly Pose**
   - Opens the chest and hips, promoting relaxation.
   - Lie on your back, bring the soles of your feet together, and let your knees fall open. Use pillows for support if needed.
3. **Legs-Up-the-Wall Pose (Viparita Karani)**
   - Relieves fatigue and promotes circulation.
   - Lie on your back with your legs extended up against a wall, arms relaxed by your sides.
4. **Supported Reclining Pose**
   - Uses bolsters or pillows to gently stretch your chest and abdomen.

How Often? Aim for 10–20 minutes a day. Over time, you'll notice better flexibility, improved sleep, and a calmer mind.

2. Community and Support: Finding Strength Together

Healing isn't meant to be done alone. Building a supportive community can make all the difference.

- **Local Support Groups**: Find groups through your cancer center or hospital. Sharing stories and advice can be deeply healing.
- **Online Communities**: Platforms like Facebook or forums connect you with women worldwide, offering support at any time.
- **Creative Outlets**: Journaling, art therapy, or even joining a book club can be therapeutic ways to connect with others and express yourself.

Gentle Reminder: Leaning on others doesn't make you weak —it highlights your courage and willingness to heal.

3. Celebrating Resilience: Honoring Your Journey

Recovery is a triumph, and every step forward deserves recognition.

- **Create Rituals**: Light a candle, plant a flower, or write a letter to your past self, honoring your strength and growth.
- **Share Your Story**: Inspire others by sharing your experience through blogs, social media, or conversations. You never know who might find strength in your words.
- **Focus on Joy**: Rediscover happiness in small things— dance, laugh, cook, and soak in the beauty around you.

FINAL THOUGHT

Cancer may have initiated the battle, but you're the one who has fought—and continues to fight—with courage, resilience, and grace. Let this chapter of your life be a testament to your strength, a reminder of your beauty, and a celebration of the life ahead. You are not just surviving; you are thriving, and that is something truly extraordinary.

Take every moment, no matter how small, and own it. This is your journey, your triumph, and your time to shine.

CONCLUSION: A HOLISTIC PATH TO WELLNESS

Breast cancer is a journey that reminds us of life's fragility but also of its boundless strength and beauty. It's a challenge that reshapes our perspective, teaching us to value every moment, every choice, and every connection. Through prevention, early detection, and thriving beyond recovery, we have the opportunity to turn adversity into a celebration of resilience and renewal.

Wellness isn't just about surviving—it's about thriving. By embracing holistic practices, we nourish our bodies with wholesome foods, move with purpose, calm our minds with mindfulness, and foster meaningful connections. Early detection becomes a gift of time and possibility, empowering us to take control of our health and the future we envision for ourselves and our loved ones.

As you walk this path, remember these words:

"Hope is not just the belief in brighter days ahead; it is the strength to create them from where we stand."

You have the power to face every challenge with grace, to turn pain into progress, and to inspire others with your courage. Your journey is not only a testament to survival but also a beacon of what it means to live fully, vibrantly, and intentionally.

Let this chapter be your reminder that your health is your most valuable asset, and your voice is your most powerful advocate. You are capable of rewriting your story, embracing each moment with an open heart, and stepping into life's next chapter with strength, hope, and joy.

CHAPTER 22

VAGINAL HEALTH AND CERVICAL CANCER

EVERYTHING YOU NEED TO KNOW TO PROTECT AND NURTURE YOUR FEMININE HEALTH

BREAKING THE SILENCE ON VAGINAL HEALTH

As women, we often carry the world on our shoulders—nurturing families, leading careers, and chasing dreams. Amid these roles, it's easy to sideline our own needs, brushing off discomfort as unimportant or too personal to address. I've seen this pattern not only in my professional life as a nurse but also in my own journey. It's not weakness that keeps us silent; it's the quiet strength of women who endure, often putting themselves last.

Let's be real—vaginal health isn't the most comfortable dinner table topic. For many of us, it's something we hesitate to bring up, whether it's out of embarrassment or fear of being dismissed. But here's the truth: your health, every part of it, deserves attention. This isn't just about easing discomfort or treating temporary symptoms; it's about prevention, awareness, and embracing the power of self-care.

Growing up in a developing country, I witnessed firsthand the devastating consequences of silence. I've heard too many stories of women suffering quietly, their symptoms dismissed as minor inconveniences until it was too late. By the time they sought help, their pain was often unbearable, and in some heartbreaking cases, their lives were already slipping away.

One memory still haunts me—a young woman in her early thirties, holding my hand as she faced the inevitable. She wasn't just a patient; she was a daughter, a sister, a mother. Cervical cancer had stolen her future, and her diagnosis came too late for intervention. That moment was a defining one for me—not as a nurse, but as a fellow woman. It reminded me that silence is not an option, and ignorance can be fatal.

Talking about vaginal health and cervical cancer may feel awkward, but these conversations are lifesaving. The power of education and awareness cannot be overstated. Understanding your body, recognizing changes, and knowing when to seek help is not just empowering—it's essential.

This chapter is a space for honesty and empowerment. It's a reminder that your health is worth prioritizing, your voice is worth being heard, and no topic is too sensitive when it comes to your well-being. Together, let's break the silence and normalize the conversation around vaginal health and cervical cancer. You deserve to thrive, not just survive—and that starts with unapologetically caring for yourself.

1. Decoding Vaginal Health: Why Awareness Is Your Superpower

The vagina is nothing short of remarkable—a finely tuned, self-regulating ecosystem that deserves admiration. At its core is a dynamic microbiome teeming with beneficial bacteria, led by the all-star **Lactobacillus**. These bacteria don't just coexist—they work tirelessly to maintain an acidic environment, with a pH delicately hovering between 3.8 and 4.5. This acidity is your body's frontline defense, fending off harmful microbes and keeping yeast at bay.

But as resilient as this system is, it's not impervious. Life has a way of shaking up this balance. Hormonal fluctuations, stress, diet, or something as seemingly benign as antibiotics can disrupt the delicate harmony. I'll never forget the time I took antibiotics for a simple dental infection, thinking little of it—until I found myself facing relentless itchiness and discomfort. That moment was a wake-up call, teaching me just how interconnected our health truly is. Even a small shift in one area of our body can ripple through others, leaving us with symptoms we didn't expect.

When you understand the intricate mechanisms behind vaginal health, it becomes more than biology—it's empowerment. Recognizing how your choices, from the foods you eat to the products you use, impact this vital ecosystem gives you the tools to safeguard your well-being.

2. Identifying a Healthy Vagina: What to Look For

A healthy vagina isn't complicated—it's beautifully straightforward when you know the signs. Here's what to expect:

- **A natural, mild odor.** Forget the myths of needing to be "odorless." Your vagina has its own unique scent, and that's perfectly normal.
- **Clear or milky white discharge.** This is a sign of a well-functioning system, acting as a natural cleanser.
- **No persistent discomfort.** Burning, itching, or irritation are signals that something's off.

Changes in any of these areas—whether it's a stronger odor, unusual discharge, or persistent discomfort—are worth paying attention to. Think of these shifts as your body's way of sending you a memo. Ignoring them is like skipping a maintenance check on a high-performance vehicle.

By embracing awareness and being attuned to your body's natural rhythms, you're not just reacting to changes—you're taking proactive steps to nurture yourself. After all, your vaginal health is an integral part of your overall wellness, and recognizing its importance is a profound act of self-care.

COMMON VAGINAL HEALTH CONCERNS AND SOLUTIONS

1. Vaginal Itchiness

- **Causes:** Common causes include yeast infections, bacterial imbalances, hormonal changes, or irritation from products like scented soaps or tight clothing.
- **Solutions:** Use antifungal creams or probiotics for yeast infections. Avoid irritants like scented products, wear breathable cotton underwear, and practice proper hygiene. Persistent or severe symptoms may require medical evaluation for tailored treatment.

2. Bacterial Vaginosis (BV)

- **Causes:** An overgrowth of harmful bacteria is disrupting the natural balance.
- **Solutions:** Antibiotics prescribed by a doctor. Prevent recurrence by avoiding scented soaps and douches.

3. Vaginal Dryness

- **Causes:** Menopause, breastfeeding, or certain medications.
- **Solutions:** Water-based lubricants or vaginal moisturizers can help. Stay hydrated and eat foods rich in omega-3s, like walnuts or flaxseeds.

4. Urinary Tract Infections (UTIs)

- **Prevention:** Stay hydrated, urinate after intercourse, and wipe front to back. Cranberry supplements can also reduce UTI risk.

COMPLETE GUIDE: HOME REMEDIES FOR VAGINAL ITCHINESS AND DISCOMFORT

Vaginal itchiness and discomfort can be uncomfortable and distracting, but they are often treatable with simple, safe home remedies and lifestyle adjustments. It's important to address the underlying causes, which may include yeast infections, bacterial imbalances, hormonal changes, allergic reactions, or irritation from fabrics or personal care products. Below is a comprehensive guide combining evidence-based natural remedies and practical advice to help alleviate symptoms and support overall vaginal health.

Probiotics and a Balanced Diet

- **Why It Works**: Probiotics help restore a healthy vaginal microbiome by promoting beneficial bacteria like *Lactobacillus*, reducing yeast overgrowth, and balancing pH levels.
- **How to Use**:
    - Incorporate probiotic-rich foods such as plain yogurt with live cultures, kefir, and fermented foods like sauerkraut into your diet.
    - Consider probiotic supplements specifically formulated for women's health.
    - Stay hydrated and eat a nutrient-rich diet with vitamins C and E, zinc, and omega-3 fatty acids to boost overall vaginal health.

Coconut Oil

- **Why It Works**: Coconut oil's natural antifungal and soothing properties help relieve irritation caused by yeast infections or dryness.
- **How to Use**:
    - Use organic, cold-pressed coconut oil. Apply a small amount externally to the affected area.

  - Avoid internal use unless recommended by a healthcare provider.

Apple Cider Vinegar Soaks

- **Why It Works**: The antimicrobial properties of raw, unfiltered apple cider vinegar can help balance vaginal pH and reduce yeast or bacterial overgrowth.
- **How to Use**:
  - Add 1–2 cups of apple cider vinegar to a lukewarm bath and soak for 10–15 minutes.
  - Avoid applying undiluted vinegar directly to sensitive areas.

Baking Soda Baths

- **Why It Works**: Baking soda restores pH balance and soothes irritation.
- **How to Use**:
  - Add 1/4 cup of baking soda to a warm bath and soak for 15–20 minutes.
  - Pat the area dry thoroughly afterward to prevent moisture buildup.

Aloe Vera Gel

- **Why It Works**: Aloe vera provides immediate relief from itching with its cooling and anti-inflammatory properties.
- **How to Use**:
  - Apply pure aloe vera gel (free of added fragrances or alcohol) externally to soothe the area.
  - Repeat as needed for ongoing relief.

Calendula

- **Why It Works**: Known for its healing and calming

properties, calendula helps reduce inflammation and irritation.
- **How to Use**:
  - Brew calendula tea, let it cool, and use it as a gentle wash.
  - Alternatively, soak a clean cloth in the tea and apply it as a compress to the affected area.

Cotton Underwear and Breathable Clothing

- **Why It Works**: Tight or synthetic fabrics can trap moisture and heat, creating a breeding ground for yeast and bacteria.
- **How to Use**:
  - Wear breathable cotton underwear.
  - Avoid tight-fitting clothing and promptly change out of wet or sweaty garments.

Cold Compresses

- **Why It Works**: Cold compresses can reduce itching, swelling, and discomfort.
- **How to Use**:
  - Wrap an ice pack in a clean cloth and apply externally for 5–10 minutes to the affected area.
  - Repeat as needed for temporary relief.

Avoiding Irritants

- **Why It Works**: Fragranced soaps, bubble baths, and douching can disrupt the natural pH of the vagina, leading to irritation.
- **How to Use**:
  - Clean the external genital area with unscented, gentle soap and warm water.
  - Avoid using douches, scented sanitary products, or harsh detergents on undergarments.

Tea Tree Oil

- **Why It Works**: Tea tree oil has natural antifungal and antibacterial properties.
- **How to Use**:
  - Dilute a few drops of tea tree oil in a carrier oil (such as coconut oil) and apply externally to relieve itchiness.
  - Use with caution as undiluted tea tree oil can cause irritation.

Boric Acid Suppositories

- **Why It Works**: Boric acid is effective for chronic yeast infections and balancing vaginal pH.
- **How to Use**:
  - Insert boric acid suppositories into the vagina as directed. These are available over the counter but should not be used during pregnancy or without medical advice.

Hydration and Proper Hygiene

- **Why It Works**: Staying hydrated promotes overall health, while good hygiene prevents infections.
- **How to Use**:
  - Drink plenty of water daily.
  - Wash the vulva gently with water and pat dry. Avoid overwashing, which can strip natural oils.

When to Seek Medical Advice

Home remedies can often provide relief, but professional medical care is crucial if:

- Symptoms persist for more than a few days or worsen.
- You experience unusual discharge, a foul odor, swelling, or severe pain.

- Over-the-counter treatments fail to improve symptoms.

FINAL THOUGHTS

Combining these remedies with good hygiene practices, a balanced diet, and lifestyle adjustments can alleviate vaginal itchiness and discomfort while promoting long-term vaginal health. Always listen to your body and consult a healthcare provider if symptoms persist or worsen.

CERVICAL CANCER: A SILENT THREAT

When we talk about women's health, breast cancer often dominates the spotlight. Yet cervical cancer, though less discussed, deserves equal attention. It's often called a "silent threat" because the early stages rarely show symptoms. The key to combating it? Prevention and early detection.

Understanding the Link to HPV

Cervical cancer is strongly linked to the human papillomavirus (HPV), a common virus most sexually active people are exposed to. While the immune system clears most infections, certain high-risk strains can lead to changes in cervical cells. Over time, these changes may develop into cancer if not caught early.

Early Detection Saves Lives

- **Routine Screenings**: Regular Pap smears and HPV tests are vital. These simple procedures can detect abnormal cell changes in the cervix before they progress.
- **Know the Warning Signs**: Be alert to symptoms like abnormal bleeding, persistent pelvic pain, or unusual vaginal discharge. These signs may seem

minor but should always prompt a visit to your healthcare provider.

A Personal Connection

A family story that stays with me is of my nanny, who lost her sister to cervical cancer. It wasn't just the loss that was heartbreaking—it was knowing that her death could have been prevented with earlier detection. This experience underlines why raising awareness about cervical cancer screenings is so essential.

Prevention is Power

- **Vaccination**: The HPV vaccine is a safe, effective way to protect against the most dangerous strains of the virus. Even adults can benefit if they haven't received the vaccine earlier in life.
- **Lifestyle Choices**: Maintaining a strong immune system helps your body naturally manage HPV infections. A healthy diet, stress management, and avoiding smoking all contribute to better cervical health.

Daily Habits for Vaginal and Cervical Health

Good habits can create a foundation for both vaginal and cervical health. These simple, consistent practices can make a significant difference:

1. Gentle Hygiene

- Cleanse the external genital area with warm water and a mild, fragrance-free soap. Avoid overwashing, which can strip natural protective oils.
- Choose breathable cotton underwear and avoid fabrics that trap moisture.

- Douches and scented feminine products are not your friends—they can upset the natural pH balance.

2. Nourish From Within

- Incorporate probiotics, such as yogurt or fermented foods, into your diet. These support a healthy vaginal microbiome and can reduce the risk of infections.
- Add colorful fruits and vegetables rich in antioxidants to strengthen your immune system and support tissue health.
- Drink plenty of water to maintain hydration and overall wellness.

3. Manage Stress for Hormonal Balance

Chronic stress disrupts hormone levels, which can affect vaginal and cervical health. Even small moments of mindfulness can help:

- Practice yoga or meditation for relaxation.
- Try journaling to process your thoughts and relieve mental strain.

4. Supporting Wellness During Vaginal Health Challenges

Challenges like vaginal itchiness, dryness, or discomfort can be frustrating, but holistic approaches can provide relief and promote long-term health.

5. Natural Relief

- **For Itchiness**: Soothing remedies like aloe vera gel or coconut oil can calm irritation.
- **For Dryness**: Opt for natural lubricants such as olive or coconut oil, especially during hormonal changes.

6. Mind-Body Connection

- Engage in deep breathing or mindfulness exercises to reduce stress-related symptoms.
- Gentle movement, like restorative yoga, can improve circulation and support relaxation.

Open Conversations Break Barriers

Talking openly with healthcare providers about your symptoms is empowering. Conversations with loved ones can also help reduce stigma, creating a supportive environment for discussing women's health issues.

CONCLUSION: EMPOWER YOUR WELLNESS JOURNEY

Vaginal and cervical health is not just a subject to approach with caution or whispers—it's a vital aspect of our overall well-being and a testament to how much we value ourselves. When we understand the remarkable balance within our bodies, embrace the power of prevention, and recognize the signals our bodies send, we're not just maintaining health; we're fostering self-respect, resilience, and empowerment.

This journey is about more than addressing discomfort or preventing illness—it's about celebrating the intricate strength and complexity of our bodies. By prioritizing our health, we're taking bold steps toward self-care and encouraging a broader culture of wellness and awareness.

WHY THIS MATTERS

Every decision you make—from the nutrients you consume to scheduling routine screenings—has a lasting impact on your well-being. These actions go beyond safeguarding yourself; they set an example for the women around you, breaking stigmas and inspiring others to prioritize their health. Whether it's addressing a persistent itch, scheduling a Pap smear, or discussing HPV prevention, each step is a declaration of self-love and proactive care.

LET'S KEEP THE CONVERSATION GOING

Knowledge becomes powerful when it's shared. Talk openly with your friends, daughters, and the women in your life about vaginal health, cervical screenings, and HPV prevention. These are not just "personal issues"—they are universal, essential parts of living vibrant, healthy lives. By normalizing these conversations, we create a culture of empowerment where no woman feels ashamed to advocate for her health.

A FINAL THOUGHT

"Awareness is the first step toward prevention, and prevention is the gift we give ourselves and future generations."

By taking charge of your health, you're not only honoring your body but also contributing to a legacy of strength and wellness. Together, we can shift the narrative from one of silence and stigma to one of courage, compassion, and celebration.

Let's move forward with confidence and commitment, embracing the power of prevention and the beauty of being informed. Together, we're not just taking care of ourselves—we're paving the way for a healthier, more empowered future for all women.

ABOUT THE AUTHOR

Hang Hoang, a resilient Vietnamese immigrant who rose above poverty and societal judgment, is a registered nurse with a Master of Science in Nursing, an Advanced Holistic Nurse Board Certification, and a Public Health Nurse Certificate. With over 16 years of dedicated practice, she is also a proud wife and mother of three young children. Crowned Mrs. Earth California 2022, Hang has been a passionate advocate for health and beauty, blending science and compassion to empower women to feel confident and radiant in their own skin. As a longtime Legislative Ambassador for the American Cancer Society, she has championed the cause of health and wellness for all. In her book, Hang shares her heartfelt journey and expert insights, offering a powerful guide for women to rediscover their glow, embrace self-care, and transform their lives from the inside out.

www.ingramcontent.com/pod-product-compliance
Lightning Source LLC
Chambersburg PA
CBHW051502150726
47997CB00001B/83